WANDER TO WONDER

My Discovery of Medical Qi Gong

Ils Cools

Countless Words

Count Less

Than the Silent Balance

Between Yin and Yang

Lao Tzu

CONTENTS

INTRODUCTION

The book you're holding came to life because of a casual remark of one of my blog readers and ex collegue. "You should make a book of all your adventures." she said. At first I discarded the idea but a seed was planted and the result you are holding in your hands or reading on your screen. The book is a compilation of blog posts that I wrote on onderwegnaaryoga.wordpress.com between November 2013 and September 2017 knitted together with some extra background, anecdotes and comments. You can recognise the blog posts by its big bold starting letter. Some of them I copied completely, some are slightly adjusted, from others I deleted parts which I found irrelevant for the story or I put them together to form a whole. I only used the ones that I found worth it, many I discarded. The ones I discarded, are posts that describe my travels and my social life and have nothing to do with Qi Gong. I didn't want to share my travel experiences with you, you can find hundreds of book on that. Neither did I want to share my social life here. You can go on Facebook for that. I wanted to share my path to the discovery of Qi Gong and the practice of it. A part of it is traveling which I didn't want to leave out because during that time, there were moments of shifting perception only to be recognised afterwards. I feel that my experience with Qi Gong can help students who start this practice. Not by searching for the same sensations as I felt but by showing them that whatever sensations they feel is perfectly normal. Many times I have been inspired by stories of senior students. Sometimes you just need to hear : "Hey I know what you feel, I went through the same." to be able to continue. During my training period in Thailand I saw many people come, go and return. I saw them struggling with the same things I was struggling with in those first months. I saw the wonder in their eyes when things started to change. I saw bodies changing, I saw minds changing. All emotions you experience during daily life, you will also experience during your practice. Anger, sadness, fear, joy, wonder, acceptance etc. All is there. How do you deal with that? By rereading what I wrote I noticed that I was holding back on the emotional stuff. I guess that was my way of dealing with it. However, you will notice that there is more lightheartedness in the writings with passing time. Again an effect of Qi Gong. Life is pretty much one big party, you don't need to take things so seriously. Shit happens, but you need shit to grow flowers. The most beautiful lotus flowers have their roots deep in the mud. Shit can also happen when English is not your mother tongue and you are translating and self publishing a book in it. This is my chance to apologise for any language mistakes. I do hope that in spite of them the underlying meaning is transfered.

◆ ◆ ◆

My Qi Gong adventures are still continuing. Curious if Qi Gong is something for you? Or do you want, just like me, more? That's possible! On www.qiflowqigong.com or www.facebook.com/qigonginsitia you can find the classes I offer. Through the contact page you can inquire about private classes or longterm arrangements.

Thank you and enjoy reading!
Ils

PART I

The Wander to Qi Gong

About yoga and travelling

(Nov 2013- Jun 2014)

1. THE BEGINNING

One drizzly morning I woke up with her words in my head: "You should make a book of it." I savoured the words and thought: "Yeah, why not? Maybe it's not a bad idea." After some doubting: "Who will want to read that? How and where to begin? Nah, I'd better occupy myself with more useful things." I put that crazy idea on hold, pulled the blankets a bit closer and snoozed a bit longer while outside the sun had difficulties to peek through the clouds. We are writing December 6, 2018, Sitia, Crete.

That same day, late in the morning, I sat behind my laptop and started typing. While in Belgium and Holland good kids got toys, chocolate figurines and mandarins for the yearly celebration of Sinterklaas, that same holy man brought me the irresistible urge to put black letters on white paper. So that's how you begin! But what was the real beginning? Friends sometimes tell me that my life resembles the life of the lady of Eat, Pray, Love. The only resemblance I see is that we both went to Asia and that that experience changed our lives. But the real beginning isn't in Asia. The real beginning is in Belgium. It all started with two independent decisions. The first one was that I would take a sabbatical year and would join a yoga teacher training course in Thailand.

How on earth did that happen? Why a TTC yoga and why Thailand? Well, it didn't happen overnight, it was a process. First there was the experience of teaching bodybalance and bodypump in a fitness center. I loved it, I was good at it (my own words...) and the feedback I got from my "students" was fantastic. What I didn't like so much was that I needed to learn the classes by means of video. What I didn't like either was the fact that I didn't have a clue what to tell people with back, neck or other problems except that they should listen to their body and not do anything that was hurting them. A bit more background would have been very useful. When the combination of teaching, work and other activities was no longer feasible, I decided I wanted to start yoga because that was the part of the classes I myself enjoyed the most. I tried different studios and found Gwenda. She works a lot with energy which appealed to me. The practice made me feel good, physically and mentally. However, I was only able to take one class a week. I wanted to start practicing on my own but there you have it. How do you start? Is there a sequence you need to follow? Can you make mistakes? This pose works with this kind of energy, that one with another kind, can they cancel each other? Will I be doing crazy things? A bit more background would have been very useful. Do you see the pattern? The search for possibilities to get that coveted background all led to one point: A teacher training course. And because of the positive experience of teaching in the fitness center, it didn't sound too crazy of an idea. So once I got my head around it I decided I wanted a real training. One that would go deep. However, none was available in Belgium or in the Netherlands. I needed to go abroad where they offer trainings from 1 to 3 months. Why eventually Thailand? Because that's where Gwenda learned her yoga and I like her style of teaching. I enrolled in June 2013 and got the final go in August 2013 together with 21 others.

The second decision was a wedding. My former partner and I decided to get married after a 12 year relationship. Both decisions started to intertwine once they were taken. The yoga TTC could only start after the wedding as to not have to organise everything at the same time. After all, the intention was for me to do the 3 month TTC after which we would travel together through Asia for about six months to end up in Crete, to find out if we could set up a bed and breakfast-yoga combination. Things went a bit different than planned. The quote "Life is what happens when you're making other plans" is definitely applicable here. Life certainly had something different in mind for the both of us. And for that to happen, my world as I knew it and cherished had to fall apart in a million pieces. One sentence brought out the first cracks.

"I don't know anymore what I feel for you. I think we shouldn't have married."

Crack, crack, craaaaack. Now what? The pieces stuck together six more weeks before they fell to my feet with one well-aimed hit.

"I want us to go our separate ways."

Only a few minutes later it hit me and tears started to flow. Tears which seemed to come out of an inexhaustible source. They appeared at the most inconvenient times. In the car while driving to work (pulling aside for a moment) at a party, while talking to a customer, in yoga class, ... Difficult moments but almost unnoticed a kind of tenacity crept in. An I-will-survive-I'm-not-going-to-cry-in-a-corner attitude. The tears dried and the preparations for the TTC could start. The fact that I was registered and the deposit was already payed gave my the power to move on. I wasn't going to let a stupid break up ruin everything. And not only that, so many people helped me through this dark period of my life. The conversations, the parties, the understanding, the encouragement, the support, everything I needed was there. You were there! Thank you! When I look back now, I can only be grateful. I wouldn't change a thing about it. I'm so happy my world has crumbled. A new and better world came to replace it. But didn't you dare tell me that while I was in the middle of it. I would not have believed you and if stares could kill, you would probably have been dead.

Although I didn't knew it back then, the most improbable and the most adventurous period of my life was about to begin.

2. PREPARATIONS

January 2, 2014, the big day, the day that I would leave Belgium for a year. Closing the door behind you and boarding the plane is the image you would see in a movie. In real life things are a bit different. You need to fill in forms for sabbatical leave, apply for a visa, get vaccinations, do your payments, make and cross to do lists, buy a phone and a laptop, pack your backpack and keep your nerves in check. I wrote it back then like this:

The first step was to put a date on my "yoga-learning" dream. When it became clear that it would be January 2014, the planning of the second step could begin: request sabbatical leave. Dilemma! How and when do you inform your employer? Officially, you only have to request it in writing maximum 3 months in advance. But in writing? And so short before leaving? No, that didn't feel right. I wanted to tell it in person and not put my employer to the brunt. Three months to find a solution for someone who wants a sabbatical year, is very short. On the other hand, how are they going to react if I communicate it too early? In these times of crisis are they not going to keep an even closer eye on me? Questions, questions, questions. That opinions in my environment differed didn't help me either. From "No, absolutely do not tell it before the official three months" to "as soon as you made your decision let them know". Eventually I followed my intuition and communicated it at a time that seemed appropriate to me. Somewhere between the two extremes, when my training application was submitted. Then I knew for sure, whatever happens, I will continue with this. Whether my employer would take it well or badly did not really matter anymore at that moment. For some it came as a surprise, others I had already informed. My employer responded positively and wished me good luck. Now I have 13 months to charge my batteries and afterwards I can just go back to work. Or maybe not. You never know what comes your way. If there is one thing that I learned in the year 2013, it is that there are no certainties in life. That everything goes by.

"Or maybe not, you never know what is coming your way." Even back then there was something inside of me that said I would not return to the job I left behind. That I would also leave the yoga behind me, I could not imagine. But first let's go back to the preparations.

Yes, I got it, my visa. Piece of cake. Fill out a 1 page form in double, add three passports photos and a copy of your flight ticket, take your passport, go to the Thai consulate on Monday, pay 60 euros and get your visa on Friday. Simple. Also the vaccinations went smoothly. On 11/12/13 (That date!) I had the last 2 of 5 injections and voilà, I am vaccinated against rabies and Japanese encephalitis. Fortunately for my poor left arm, I was already vaccinated against hepatitis A and B, typhoid fever and yellow fever.

The payment of the training took a lot more effort and therefore my mind was already making up all kinds of doomsday scenarios. The most common was the one in which I could not participate. By now, I know that if it is meant for you, it will come. If not, then not. In both cases worrying and imagining the worst are only a waste of time and energy. After 5 attempts and a few times driving back and forth to the bank I could put my mind at ease. The payment was successful. The purchase of a laptop and a phone was a whole other story which left me with quite a few sleepless nights. After all, your first smartphone is something so important that you need to surf to

700 comparison sites and loose your sleep while your brain keeps firing RAM and GB numbers to get you even more confused. Admittedly, it has been useful because on that same laptop, I now type these words. The smartphone didn't last that long. Besides all that, there was this:

In between buying presents, celebrating Christmas and New Year and visiting all the people who would like to say goodbye before leaving, I have to get passport pictures, go to the hairdresser, return my library books (No, Ils, don't bring any new ones! That fine is really going to be too high!) and buy half a pharmacy worth of pills. Well, that's how I see it anyway. I may have a degree which states that I am a pharmacist, at home I only have something for an upset stomach and a painkiller, probably 7 years passed expiry date. Just saying that I rarely take medicines and that the quantities that are now in front of me are more than everything I have taken in the last 15 years. Meanwhile, almost everyone asks if my suitcase is ready. Uhm. No. I'm too busy with buying presents, eating out, marking off to-do lists and so on. I think I've got everything I need, but packing will be done the evening of January 1. And it is not a suitcase but a backpack. I hope that I can keep the weight below 15kg, preferably around 10kg. For those who are horrified by the idea of having only 2 panties, I assume that you may double that number for thongs. With these wise words, I want to conclude and I wish you all happy holidays. The next post will be from the other side of the world! I'm practically bouncing off the walls!

Yes, I was bouncing off the walls but I was also scared. I was wondering whether this was the right choice, whether I would manage travelling by myself. Would I be safe? Wouldn't I be lonely? Those feelings the last days before my departure. Swinging from ecstatic to depressed and back. From Bangkok it sounded much more subdued:

First I should say something about the last days in Belgium. Packing my backpack was a disillusionment. I really thought I had packed very limited. The first weighing turned out I was grossly mistaken: 18kg! Alas, those pants, that t-shirt and those beauty creams have to stay home. I will wear that top and leave that one at home. This travel guide? Nope, no can take. The verdict: 2.3kg less! Still too much but it will have to do. January 1 was a difficult day. Finishing some last little things and then there was a lot of time to think. I was already tearing up and receiving some heartfelt text messages made it even worse. Fortunately, January 2 was better. Saying goodbye at the airport is not fun, but we all know that it is only for three months. In April mom, dad, brother and his girlfriend are coming to visit me.

The flight to Bangkok with a stopover in Doha was in my eyes very luxurious. A whole multimedia library for yourself? Wow great! By now I don't expect anything less! We are so easily spoiled, aren't we? Anyway, my favorite activity during long haul flights is still watching cartoons. That habit started back then.

The first part of the flight to Doha was nice, no turbulence and all the luxuries you can imagine. As most of my friends know, I don't have a TV at home but I am a fan of cartoons. And guess what, I could watch them on my private screen. I made up for my loss: three cartoons (or are they called animation movies now?), one after the other. The second part, from Doha to Bangkok, I wanted to sleep but some newborns had others ideas. Row 10 was the baby row with three babies next to each other and who was sitting just behind it? In row 11? Yep. And it was as if they had agreed not to cry at the same time but one after the other. I arrived in Bangkok with big black bags under my eyes, looking very pretty, ahum. Got hold to Thai Baht and a Thai Sim Card very easily.

Taking the train to the center was no problem either. I took a tuk-tuk from the station to Khao San road and haggled down the price from 200 to 100 baht. I wonder if that was still a rip-off. I also quickly got a ticket for Koh Phangan, my destination for the next 12 weeks.

Everything and everyone is quite relaxed here. The same goes for me after my first Thai shoulder, neck and back massage. Never thought that such a delicate Thai lady had so much power in her hands. Goose bumps all over my body, ending with a loud crack when she practically wrung me out. But I feel loose now. I also visited my first temple. People still crawl on their knees for the monks here. First they donate their offerings and afterwards they chant together. Nice to watch but to participate? No, not really my cup of tea. I wasn't even supposed to be there, I had hidden myself in the back because I was not allowed inside with my shorts and strap top. All these impressions made my stomach grumble. So I picked up a delicious padthai prepared by a very friendly lady for only 25 Baht or 60 euro cent!

What I did not mention in that post was my very first experience with Thai cuisine: Tom Yam or spicy lemongrass soup. Tom Yam has lemongrass and galangal, in addition to some other ingredients. And it was the galangal that has spoiled my view of Tom Yam soup for a long time. Galangal is a root that looks a bit like ginger and that you don't eat. It's added to the soup for the taste. A taste that is somewhat like ginger but a lot stronger. I speak from experience because I took that piece of galangal in my mouth and bit on it. And spit it out again. Ugh! Suddenly I was not hungry anymore. The padthai later was a safer choice! Traveling alone as a woman is also very safe in Asia. I really shouldn't have worried. I was not the only one who traveled alone and it seemed that like-minded people attract each other. I didn't lack company or conversation. Neither on my way to Koh Phangan nor on later travels.

3. TTC YOGA

When I think back to the TTC yoga it is as if it never happened. It almost looks like I have banned that time from my memory. Only by reading again what I wrote back then, the memories surface. Those memories are more about what happened besides the TTC than about the TTC itself. The sessions with Taro for example which I, for whatever reason, didn't mention in the blog posts. I think I was ashamed. Yet it has been her direct, not always gentle approach that has opened my eyes to my carefully constructed defense tactics. Defensive tactics that I used unconsciously not to face the reality of certain feelings. But let's go back to another beginning. The moment I met Taro, a Dutch lady, for the first time. It was during a dynamic meditation workshop that Gwenda, my yoga teacher, organized. I suppose I was curious and wanted to know what it was all about. I never could have imagined what an effect Taro would have on my life. I don't believe that at that moment I knew that Taro lived on Koh Phangan and was only in Belgium for a short intermezzo. What I still remember from the dynamic meditation was that I felt very uncomfortable and that Taro evoked a kind of awe. That tall

Dutch lady who had difficulties walking, who with her crooked witch fingers made fun of everything and who saw life as one big party. I will never forget the first time I visited her on Koh Phangan. She lived on my way to the yoga hall so it was only logical that I would drop by to say hello. The first thing she said to me was: "I heard from Gwenda that you split up with your husband, congratulations, you were with him for the wrong reasons." I stood there, shocked, not knowing what to say, boiling inside, thinking: "How on earth can you know that? Because of the two conversations you and I had?"

"Take a seat, dear."

"Er, yes, thank you" And I curled myself up in an armchair.

We chit chatted a bit, talked about the training and how I saw it and then suddenly she said:

"You're afraid of being here, aren't you?"

"Huh, no, no"

"Oh yes you are, I can see it."

"No, I'm not!"

She with a smile on her face: "Okay, sit like this, legs apart and hands on your knees"

With a sigh I left my curled up position and did what she asked for.

Two seconds later... "Okay, you're right. Thank you."

And I folded back into the armchair and my shell. Tjakka, defense tactic number 1 went flying out of the window. I was the first of many because although I often felt uncomfortable in her presence, there was something sincere in her way of being that fascinated me. She wouldn't let you get away with bullshit or excuses. I was not the only one who felt that way. She gave satsang every Monday and usually a group of about 7 people would attend. She talked about things like Silent Awareness, Oneness etc. Things that made little sense to me. She turned up her nose when you said you were looking for happiness. Or satisfaction. For her there was only one cause worth striving for and that was inner peace and freedom. Now I understand better what she was talking about. When you are looking for happiness or satisfaction, it means that you are pushing away a part of life. The part that shows itself to you now and that you are not satisfied or happy with. You want more, tomorrow is going to be better. But tomorrow will never come. It's like going to that bar where there is a sign saying: "Tomorrow free beer" When will you get that free beer do you think? Right, never. Likewise with happiness or satisfaction. If you push away certain emotions because you label them as bad, they continue to fester under the surface. If you, on the contrary, allow them to just be there, you will see that they have their own course. They come and they go, without you having to do anything. You can be the spectator, you are the Silent Awareness from which your whole life unfolds. You really don't have to do anything. And that, I understand now, is the peace and freedom that Taro wanted to show me and other seekers. Because that was us, the thousands of yoga students on that Thai island. Seekers. We were looking for something that we often could not name ourselves. There had to be something more in life, no? And that more yoga would give us. The crux is that nothing or nobody can give you that more. Only you can recognize that more in yourself when you take a step back and let go of the control you think you have. But let's go back to the yoga training and how I experienced that.

U nbelievable, the first week is almost over. I feel exhausted. The focus was mainly on theory and less on asanas (= exercises). We get one asana per day in the morning class. But before we get to practice we receive a lot of information about some other yoga related subject and about the asana itself. It's the other way around in the afternoon class. There we practice first and afterwards we get yoga related theory. A lot of information and on some days my head was about to burst. In addition, they say here that your body is purified by the techniques giving you a number of so-called purification reactions which include amongst other fatigue and outbursts of acne. Tell me about it! On day 4 I was so exhausted that I missed the (optional) lecture given by swami and fell into my bed at 9 o'clock! The purification acne I have too and some pain in the shoulders that they cannot explain. Exhausting.

God, yes, those purification reactions. Everything

that was out of the ordinary was called purification. An easy way to get away with anything. I don't deny that there is truth in it. Also in Medical Qi Gong it is generally accepted that the body can hold trauma and emotions. The difference is that in yoga it was seen as a sign that there is improvement happening while in Qi Gong it is seen as a symptom of where you're not balanced yet. An example to clarify it.

Yoga:

"Teacher, I have pain in my shoulders"

"Oh, don't worry, you're going through a purification phase"

Qi Gong:

"Teacher, I have pain in my shoulders"

"Yes, drop them, relax them." Or "Yes, relax and come more to the balls of your feet." Or "Yes, bring your chin back. "Or" Yes, less thinking. "

The pain in my shoulders that I felt at the time was mainly due to a wrong posture (shoulders raised and pulled back), but I only learned that a few months later when Qi Gong came into my life. For now, let's go back to the yoga. I had mixed feelings about it. On one hand I was enthusiastic, on the other hand there were doubts too.

Absolutely interesting! To learn more about the asanas, what they do, how they should be executed, how they relate to each other and to the world. More of that, please! I am already looking forward to the anatomy and physiology lessons to learn more about their effect on the body. And of course it is super interesting to learn how the asana's are just a part of the yoga system. There are other parts too. Some of these parts and theories, however, are far from what my scientific mind can understand and accept. I hear them but I have a lot of reservations about them. An example: According to the yogis (those who can know because they were enlightened and received their information from above) the body actually consists of 5 bodies: the physical body, the energetic body, the astral body, the mental body and the causal body. Everyone sees his own body so physical body: okay. Energetic body: okay because I already felt energy before I came here. And anyone who does Tai Chi or Qi Qong can confirm this. But then. The astral body allows you to be at 2 places simultaneously by means of astral projection, the same for the mental body by means of mental projection and the causal body allows you to influence events. I can still accept the latter. Most of us have already experienced that when we wanted something to happen, it actually happened. But mental and astral projection? Really? Then it happens that the next day you talk with one of your fellow students (a dentist) and it turns out that he can project himself astrally! He learned it from a book! Whaaaat ???? !!!! I guess I have to accept that there is more between heaven and earth than what I've known. True, I discover new sensations myself. I have already said that I could feel energy before I came here. Mainly between my hands and only if I really concentrate on it. I have never felt the chakras (or energy centers) though. During the yoga in Belgium I occasionally felt some heat or some tingling in my spine during certain exercises but that was it. Yesterday during the music meditation I clearly felt the 2nd, 4th and 6th chakra. Strange. And I can't explain how it feels because they all feel different. And I didn't feel them all the time, just during moments of great focus. That seems to be really crucial.

Feeling energy? Feeling Chakras? Intrinsically, there is nothing wrong with that. I suppose this was a process that I had to go through to realize afterwards that it was child's play. That much what happened back then was a mind game. Think of something long enough and you feel it. We were kind off indoctrinated by the use of standard phrases that were repeated in every class. They told us where and how the energy was flowing. In the TQH system very little to nothing is said about energy but we can see it and test if it is present. It appears and accumulates, purely because of the right posture, adopted in a state of relaxation, physically and mentally. At that moment, however, I was not yet at that point. But there was hope, I wasn't completely lost.

A ccording to a number of teachers here, most people are like sheep, they do what the masses do. The teachers call them sheeple. On the contrary, we, students of yoga and spirituality, have stepped out of that pattern by our choice to follow this path. Could be, but when I see some students here, completely going along, almost in worship, with all what is being said, I wonder where the difference is.

Indeed, from one herd to another. From the house, the big car (preferably two) and the piles of money to the best meditation, the most difficult yoga pose and the highest spiritual realization. And of course our yoga school was the best. With its video lessons which made me doze off, its laya yoga where you had to meditate for half an hour on the ringing in your ears in which, thank God, I never succeeded and a swami who asks you during a mandatory private conversation inappropriate questions about your sex life. "Hello Mr. Swami, I am here to learn yoga, my sex life, which is non-existent by the way, is none of your business." When, in response to the #metoo movement in 2018, a rather big amount of yoginis and female teachers signed an open letter with accusations of sexual abuse by Swami, I wasn't surprised at all. And then there was the ping pong ball.

The ping pong ball. I don't see it. I should see it, but I don't. It goes as follows. You hold a ping pong ball in front of you, you look at it for 30 seconds or until you think you know how it looks like. Then you close your eyes and try to get the image of that ping pong ball in front of your mind's eye. Only the ball, not the background, not the hand with which you hold it. If the image of the ping pong ball has disappeared, you open your eyes and start all over again. You do that for 5 minutes (to begin with). I do not see that stupid ball, I see all sorts of other things. Like hundreds of ping pong balls jumping out of my forehead, but I just can't picture one simple orange ping pong ball in front of my mind's eye. Frustrating.

Looking back, I wonder what the hell we were doing. There are other, more useful ways to sharpen your concentration and focus. Do a few hours of Qi Gong every day for two weeks and you will notice that your concentration and focus has improved by leaps and bounds. And on top of that you will know more about what is going on in your body. I still remember a lecture in which one of the senior teachers said that they were a bit crazy in India. Rolling from one city to another as a pilgrimage, or standing on one leg for days on end. What is the difference with trying to visualize a ping pong ball or with Trataka? Trataka is 5 minutes staring at a black dot without blinking your eyes. One, you start to see double and two, the tears run down your cheeks because your eyeballs dry out and the natural reaction of the body is to prevent that. And this should be beneficial for your eyes? Do you believe that I have my doubts? Not to mention all those crazy purification techniques such as drinking salt water on an empty stomach and puking it back out, or "purification by fire" a breathing technique that can make you faint.

I was so shocked that my body trembled for the remainder of the class! What happened? We are learning a technique that they call Agnisara Dhauti or the "purification by fire". By breathing in a certain way you are supposed to send energy from your abdominal center to your heart center. You can do the technique in three ways: sitting with your buttocks on your heels, on your knees or standing up. And this in order of strength. So if you do it standing upright, there is a lot more energy involved. The problem is to keep that energy from going to your head because it may happen that you pass out. I myself don't sense much during the exercise, so I was very sceptical. I thought it was all just blahblah. After yesterday I clearly have to reconsider. It is very frightening when you hear a thump, you look behind you and you see someone laying on the floor, unconscious, convulsing a few times with her hands still on her stomach and her chin bleeding. Two seconds later she regained her conscious. Fortunately for her she was performing the exercise on her knees. If she had been upright, it could have been much worse. I definitely have to check again what the benefits of this technique are. At the moment I have forgotten them and I wonder why they teach us something like this.

Besides the exercises that some were felled by, there was also the Thai concrete that made victims. My not so mild collision looked like this.

AAAAH, kabong, boom patat. And there we were, in a flash of a second, stretched out on the Thai concrete. Fortunately nothing serious except what ugly looking and painful abrasions for me and a small fracture in the foot for my driver. All that because a dog who wanted to commit suicide. He suddenly came running out of the bushes and hits the front wheel of our motorcycle. We topple over and glide on our side over the Thai roads. And that exactly three days before I move closer to the yoga hall and no longer have the need for a motorcycle. Karma? It certainly is a bitch. However, it could have been much worse. Oh yeah, the dog? He's fine.

Not everything was so dramatic. There were also many instructive and fun moments. Like these two. Totally unrelated though.

I loved the talks about detachment and satisfaction. Detachment means that you can have everything (money, a house, friendships, relationships, ...) but that from one moment to the next you have to be able to leave everything behind without any drama. That you know that nothing is yours, that you don't own anything. Like people, they just can disappear from your life one day and that's okay. I think it's a beautiful concept but live it? That seems to be a whole other story to me! Satisfaction sounds easy but it's not. Can you be as satisfied with the good things as with the 'bad' things that happen to you? Can you accept everything that happens to you with gratitude and see the good in it? Also the difficult and not so nice circumstances? Satisfaction and detachment are connected, because how can you be satisfied when you lose stuff and people that you are attached to? And yet detachment is not equal to indifference. Something to think about.

Yesterday I snorkeled for the first time. Amazing!!! In the beginning it took a bit to get used to blowing the water out of the snorkel but once I got the trick it was great. Relaxing, almost like a meditation. And what a beautiful world, that underwater world! Beautiful colored corals, magnificent fish. So many different kinds: zebrafish, fluorescent fish, translucent fish, black fish and so much more. At one point we were completely surrounded by a school of fish. Indescribable, time stood still. But above the water the world was turning as usual. It had started to rain and it was a lot colder when we finally emerged. But I enjoyed it immensely! Thank you Kate for teaching me how to snorkel!

And that was it from Koh Phangan. I went back once, for a week, about 7 months later. Not to do yoga, but to visit Taro and to inhale the fresh sea air. My last musings about the TTC:

Wow, finished! Twelve weeks passed by, it's hard to believe. It went so fast! It has been quite an experience and I am no longer the Ils who left Belgium three months ago. I notice that my happiness is much less dependent on the outside world. Thanks to the combination of working with Taro and doing yoga, I have discovered a place within myself where it is always quiet, where everything is good no matter what happens around me. It is a source of wellbeing that does not depend on what I think about myself, on what I think others think about me or on the circumstance, whether good or bad. That place, that source is always here, I can always access it. It is very easy to get there. One exhale and one step back. Taking that step back is simple. Becoming aware of the fact that I am completely carried away by what is going on, that's the difficult part. Once I am aware: Ooh, I am doing it again, I am back in the "I cannot do this" role, or in the "I don't feel like it" role or in the "No, I cannot cry/be angry/be afraid because what will they think of me "role or in the" I have to plan everything "role, the step back is almost done. It's a matter of experiencing that life has so much beauty to offer if you don't fight it. Like this last week. I had an image, a plan in my mind how it should be. It turned out to a bit differently. For once I listened to my intuition. It brought me a lift to Thongsala, a bikini for 30 baht (less than a euro), a skipped practicum that turned out to be so bad I didn't miss anything and a lot of wisdom! I passed my exams and I got that much coveted certificate. The strange thing is that it doesn't seem to matter anymore. If you have mastered something truly and completely, you can pass it on. Whether you have a piece of paper or not. When I started three months ago, that paper certificate was my goal. The next course I will no longer start with a piece of paper in mind. The questions I'll ask are: "Can it contribute to my personal growth?" and "Is it fun?" Especially the latter!

Wise words then. "If you have mastered something, you can pass it on." You do not need a certificate for that. Unfortunately, the Western world mostly disagrees and too much emphasis is placed on knowledge instead of experience. Also the TTC was mainly focused on knowledge. 500 hours of which almost half were filled with theory. In three months only 4 classes where you were to teach yourself. And that's enough to call yourself a yoga teacher? Honestly? Where is the experience? Of course back then I had a different view. I thought I knew my body, I thought I knew what was right and what was wrong, I thought I had fully mastered things. I would found out very soon I hadn't.

4. IN BETWEEN TRAVELS

The yoga TTC might have been finished and I might have been thinking that I was ready for a life as a yoga teacher, the experience taught me I was not. To be honest, during the training I already had doubts whether this was the right thing for me. I felt that my body would not be able to endure that daily torture until I retired. Whenever I did, for whatever reason, no asana's for a day, I felt stiff and sore the next day. It was like everytime I had to start all over again. I shared my concerns with a fellow student. Told her that I would like to work more with energy. Actually a combination of exercises and energy. In return, she told me about a week-long course she completed in Chiang Mai. Medical Qi Gong Level 1. She gave me the website of ThaiQiHolistics and said to give it a chance. According to her, the teacher seemed to know a lot about energy. The note with the website adress was tucked away for a later time. First there was a week in Penang, Malaysia to get used to normal life again. As if being a tourist in Georgetown can be considered as normal. Georgetown with its melting pot of cultures, its large bling bling shopping centers and its tiny, dark, filled until the ceiling curiosa shops, its little India where you are bombarded with a cacophony of sounds and smells, where from all different sides the "ohm shanti hare hare" blasts out of the speakers, not quite simultaneously nor synchronously. Where the goldsmith is already persuading you to buy while you still are kindly trying to say no to the sari tailor. Where men and women don't talk but shout in their phones. Its Chinese section with colorful temples and beautiful old buildings, its street art in hidden corners and alleys, its large mosque that determines the rhythm of daily life with the call to prayer. If you go outside the city, you will find beaches, buddhist temples and a national park where you can have nice walks and encounter some wildlife.

L ike a troop of monkeys. They were blocking the path on my way back to the entrance. I approached to about a meter. After a stand-off with a growling monkey who was showcasing his teeth for about 30 seconds, which seemed to last for an eternity and during which I was trembling on my legs, the troop decided that it was not worth to attack me. They left and I was able to continue my journey. Almost at the end of the walk I suddenly spotted a large lizard (?) swimming in the sea. I stopped walking and stood very quietly on the path hoping he would come on the beach so I could take a picture. No picture though, thanks to three English boys who saw it too and chased it like paparazzi would have chased Ed Sheeran. Of course it swims away. I would too.

Back to Thailand for example. Luckily I did not have to swim, I could just take the bus to Bangkok where I would be reunited with my parents and my brother and his girlfriend. To travel together for three weeks throughout Thailand. A little culture, some nature, a bit sporty and a bit lazy. A nice mix of everything. A severe stomach flu during the second week (39°C fever, diarrhea, sleepless nights) of which the remnants remained until two weeks later partly ruined it for me. It also meant that I was far from being pleasant company. Certainly not during the first three days when the illness was at its peak and the fever and the loss of fluid completely exhausted my body. Afterwards too, I preferred my bed and the coolness of the air conditioning over a dinner with the family. Much to their regret. A number of hard words fell and some tears flowed but the core of our conflict was not my illness or my withdrawal. The core was concern. Concern from my parents that their daughter with her three university degrees would waste her life and end up in the gutter. That she would become a stranger. They did not understand why I had chosen a different path. To be honest, at that moment I was a bit of a bitch who thought she was the sole possessor of a superior truth, who sometimes made spiteful remarks because she thought her views were so much better. Qi Gong, along with dozens of devoured spiritual books and getting older (?) has soften me alot and taught me acceptance. I will still express my opinions, but I no longer have to convert you to my view. My parents and I have traveled together for another 3 weeks twice and I think they can confirm that both times it was a much more enjoyable experience. So I did not become a stranger. They see that I am a different person, one who is much more satisfied with her life, whatever comes on her path. But that was later. First there was Thailand to explore. From Bangkok to the River Kwai, from Chiang Mai and the opium triangle to Sukothai and Khao Yai with the last stop a beach in Krabi.

I t was a happy reunion at our hotel in Bangkok where we shared the latest news over a hearty breakfast. With our bellies filled we went on our way to Wat Pho and the Grand Palace. And got caught in a travel scam. The temple would only be open in the afternoon, it was better to do a boat trip first. Only 23€ per person. Uhm, no thanks. And off course Wat Pho wasn't closed at all, neither was the Grand Palace.

We saw a different part of Bangkok during a cycling trip. You start in the posh part of Bangkok, cycle for 100m and find yourself in the slums. From there you drop the bicycle in a longboat which get you and your bicycle to the jungle. Basically it's just a kind of green space that consisted of small plantations of fruit and vegetables between the coconut, mango and papaya trees. But it did have the feel of jungle and was a nice getaway from the hustle and bustle of the city.

No cycling but walking on the famous Bridge over the River Kwai, part of the Death railway. The museum about the construction of the railway, the war cemetery and the Hell Fire Pass (a gorge that was manually excavated) left me the very strong impression that humankind is not kind at all. The night was spent on the river itself, in the Jungle Rafts Hotel. Very cool hotel, floating rafts, no electricity, everything illuminated with oil lamps, very neat. The coolest thing about the hotel was what I call bodyrafting. You put a lifejacket on, you jump in the water in front of room 1, you let yourself be carried away by the current, or swim against it if you want some training, and make sure you grab yourself onto room 63 to restart the game.

A lot of water too in our next stop, Chiang Mai. Every year somewhere in April the Thai New Year, Songkran, better known as the water festival, is celebrated. Oh dear! All streets blocked with pick up trucks from which people are throwing water on you. With buckets, spray guns or even fire hoses. Nothing to do than to grab a bucket yourself and play along. Until you get a shower with ice water. So cold! And right at that moment the sun disappeared behind the clouds. Dripping and shuddering we wisely decided we had seen enough water for that day.

The five-day tour with the minivan along Mae Hong Son, Pai, Thaton and Chiang Rai started off very well. An hour's drive to a waterfall. Blissfully soothing, the 'noise' of water. Next a walk of about 2 hours through the jungle with a local guide. Brilliant! Learning to imitate animal sounds with plants, tasting cinnamon root, smelling the tree bark which is used to make tiger balm and making shampoo from a kind of fruit. Unfortunately all good things come to an end and about halfway through the 5 hour journey I began to feel sick. My stomach was upset, I got goosebumps and chills. Yet we arrived at the hotel without accidents. I decided to skip dinner though. Good decision, the "Happy Room" (our driver's word for toilet) appreciated my company. I didn't appreciate it at all, I don't consider 39.5 degrees fever and diarrhea good company.

The next morning the rest of the family went to visit a temple and the long neck tribe while I stayed in my hotel room until they were back in the afternoon. Special arrangement made by my brother. Thank you Tim! Still 38.3 fever and diarrhea but we really had to continue our trip. Nothing to do but to take some medication and stay in the van while my family was having fun. Seat back, fan on and trying to rest because the driving did not help either. Anyone who travelled through Asia will confirm that they have a particularly crazy driving style. The night was long and I wouldn't call it restful but fortunately the fever had subsided the next morning. I managed to eat a small piece of toast just to have something in the stomach. Day 3 was waiting for us. First to a geyser. Lovely smell, a hint of rotten eggs, very pleasant if you're not fully recovered yet. And then they're going to boil eggs in it! Our driver persuaded me to eat a very small piece of egg (IL you must eat, good for stomach). Wrong move! I had to stay in the van for the rest of the day and missed all the good things. To be honest, at the time, I couldn't care less. The only thing I wanted was to recover as quickly as possible. And that seemed to happen the morning of day 4. Carefully ate one piece of French Toast with honey. It didn't want to leave my body immediately, yay, progress. I also managed to get through the tea tasting, the feeding of temple monkeys and the boat trip on the Mekong where Myanmar, Laos and Thailand are just a stone's throw from each other. Yet decided to skip dinner because the belly was still not quite as it should have been.

The last day of the tour held the highlight.

A two-hour ride on the back of an elephant. By the time I had found out how to sit without hitting my back against the iron seat, I was completely bruised. But it was a fantastic ride. Very beautiful nature, very quiet. You only heard the insects and the babbling of a brook. Even the elephants almost made no noise. Toward the end, I was allowed to come out of the seat and actually sit behind the ears. Weird feeling, not easy to keep your balance but very nice. I also had the idea that the elephants were treated well. They were not beaten up and the men seemed to have conversations with them. That can also be my imagination. Somewhere halfway through the ride, my driver asks if he should take pictures. Yes, please, ever tried to take pictures on a wobbly elephant? So he just jumps off and starts taking pictures of the whole family. My elephant quietly walking along with me, only obeying on spoken commands. Good boy, good boy. Some moments later a shrieking cry, elephant stops and driver climbs back on. Phew!

Lunch was lovely but my belly didn't like so much the padthai I had (grrrr!). Luckily we were still in the restaurant. When the bowels were happy again, we went on to the white temple in Chiang Rai. Eccentric is the least you can say. A Buddha statue on one side, murals of Michael Jackson, Kungfu

Panda, The Matrix and Avatar on the other. It was a nice conclusion to a beautiful five-day event. Too bad I missed a day and a half of it. You may wonder: "What about your yoga? Can't you do anything with it?" "Yes, but a deep massage of your stomach when it is very swollen, is not something you want to try if only putting your hands on it hurts. Let alone squeezing that belly to do a certain breathing exercise!"

By now, I learned to deal with diarrhea in a much more gentle way. A number of acupressure points can be stimulated without having to come near to your stomach. Also the Qi Gong exercises themselves are a lot gentler to do during illness. It was/is one of Ajahn's mottos. Attend class when you are sick or when you are feeling under the weather. It's then that you need Qi Gong the most. It's then that you will learn the most about your body. Unfortunately, I did not have that knowledge available when I needed it and I couldn't help my body in its healing effort. It had to do it by itself during the continuation of our Thai adventure that brought us via scorching Su-khothai with its very impressive temple complex to Khao Yai where we met a whole series of beautiful and less beautiful specimens. From a whip snake that the guide pulled from some bushes next to the road to a 25cm long millipede, a tarantula, a poisonous centipede and a scorpion spider to millions of bats that came out of their cave in one long uninterrupted wave.

We watched for forty minutes and they still kept coming! It was an incredibly beautiful spectacle! With some extra entertainment when a hawk came to pick up its dinner. On top of that, we were able to admire an owl on our way back.

Day 2 in Khao Yai was filled with searching for and admiring different species of wild-life. At the first stop we could see hornbills and macaques. During the walk that fol-lowed, we had the surprise of our lives. First we saw a chameleon. Everyone takes pic-tures (we were with a group of 9) and then we continue. We were not even ten steps further when my mum said: "Hey, come back, there is a snake here". I was right behind the guide so I passed him the information. He answers seemingly surprised: "Really?" And then sud-denly he takes action. He is practically run-ning back while calling: "Careful, careful it can be poisonous". Yes, very poisonous. The green pig viper is one of the deadliest snakes in the world. When you're bitten you have 8 hours to get to a doctor. Fortunately they are not active during the day and this little one had eaten the night before. Shown by the bulge in its body. It was just laying there on a branch of a fern. My brother had broken off the branch next to it. So the rest of the walk everyone was very careful to grab something! We also encountered Gibbons and a scorpion on that same walk. After the walk we went looking for elephants. We were fortunate enough to see a monitor lizard and macaques during the search. And elephants! Many elephants. First a solitary male and then a whole herd of about 16 animals. With a very young one that was very well protected. It was usually hidden between two large animals but occasionally we could spot it. Cute! There was another very rude animal. A Homo Sapiens who was walking alone and who had approached the elephants way too close. Our guide said that three months earlier, a European tourist was trampled by charging elephants. Some people really do everything to take the perfect picture.

After two days animal spotting, it was time to take a rest on a white beach. After a flight and a taxi ride we had to take a wooden longboat. By the time we had all the luggage on board, even our underwear was wet. Luckily, the water was warm. Which also meant that it does not really cool you down when you are sunbathing. But actually it is not safe to sunbathe, even in the shade it takes only an hour for your skin to take on a lobster like shade. To spare our skin a bit we booked a snorkel tour. It would have been more accurate to call it island sitting tour. We have snorkeled for half an hour, jumped off a cliff for 5 minutes and the rest of the time we spend on the boat or on an island. With 300 other people. All crammed together in the scarce spots of shade. And this is low season, I don't even want to think about high season! Although, if you could think away the people and the boats, we would be sitting in a beautiful, idyllic place with limestone rocks shooting straight out of the sea.

The last day together with the family was a quiet day. The night was a little less quiet. We were already used to the fact that it rained almost every night and that there were thunderstorms every now and then but that night was the worst. The first thunderbolt made me jump half a meter out of my bed. And the second one was so loud that the bed shook!

The next day was the last day of our family trip. At the airport of Krabi we all shed some tears while saying goodbye. Thank you Tim and Linde for arranging everything, thank you mum and dad for coming all the way to Thailand! It was lovely to see you again.

There I was, my backpack a bit lighter because my parents took some stuff back to Belgium but in fact it was still too heavy to be comfortable. I had two weeks to fill before traveling through Indonesia with

Mariska, a former colleague. The plan was to stay in Krabi town for a night and travel on to Koh Lanta the next morning. I ended up staying two nights in Krabi because the Tibetan Book of Living and Dying, found on the coffee table of the guesthouse, had to be finished first. Don't ask me how Krabi town looks like, I have no idea. I only emerged from the world of the book to arrange the transfer to Koh Lanta. I have never been interested in religion, still not by the way, but the death book as it is sometimes called fascinated me. It was my first encounter with a very different view on death.

I t is about how Tibetan Buddhists and ordinary Tibetan people face life and death. But mainly about how they deal with death. They say that you can only die properly if you have lived properly. And living means for them to make a connection with the divine (or whatever you want to call it) in yourself.

In our Western culture we try to avoid the subject of death to all costs, as if talking about it or thinking of it evokes the man with the scythe. Yet, the only certainty in life is that one day we will be no longer among the living. From the moment you are born you are on your way to your death. How fast or slow that day is coming, you don't know. Are you ready? Am I ready? I don't know. What I do know is that I was clearly not ready that day in the van on the way to Koh Lanta.

After half an hour drive I had to sit in front next to the driver because some other people joined us. I'd rather have been in the back after all. There you notice that they drive fast but you don't see that the meter says 120 km per hour on lanes where you can drive a maximum of 70 in Belgium. That they cross cars just before the corner or when an oncoming car is approaching and that they tail drive motorcycles. You only hear that they honk, you don't know why. I was happy when we arrived and I could get out!

I didn't have a plan really, but I ended up staying on Koh Lanta for two weeks. The first week was filled with adrenaline rushes. For the first time driving a scooter myself and that while I remembered all too well the slide we took on Koh Phangan. For the first time diving and admiring the colorful underwater world. Seeing a school of dolphins jumping up as an extra treat. For the first time getting a leech in your toe, seeing him swell and pulling him out with lots of ews. Fears were overcome, the denigrating commentator voice in my head was cut short. Woehoe!

To scooter or not to scooter? That was the question that kept me busy all day long. It accompanied me to the beach, to dinner, while watching an absolutely amazing sunset, while listening to the guitarist's performance and the corny rock songs that the Pad Thai Band, a gang of old Thai rockers, brought. To scooter won. At 20 km per hour, sometimes a bit more, cruising the east side of the island on my rented scooter. I stopped for a boat trip through the mangrove forest. The captain showed me crabs, birds and monkeys. After nature it went to a small town for some healthy fuel for myself. Old Town is a charming fishing village where Buddhists, Chinese and Muslims live together peacefully. I had a delicious vegetarian curry soup with roti there. On the way back I visited the cemetery of the sea gypsies. They bury their dead on a sand dune which is flooded so the sea takes the bones to their eternal resting place. To honor them they celebrate from morning 8 till evening 4. No sad funerals like ours. They believe that if they are happy and celebrate, their deceased are also happy and celebrate. Nice, isn't it?

The next day I drove along the west coast of Koh Lanta. I wanted to visit the Tiger Cave. The booklet about Koh Lanta said only that it was a mysterious experience. Yeah, say that again!

First obstacle: a cow and her calf. The calf loose, Ma cow tied to a pole with a rope of about three meter. The calf approaches me curiously which Ma cow didn't like at all. She started to moo and demonstratively blocked my way. I kindly asked Ma cow if I could pass. Apparently not. There I was, not knowing what to do, meanwhile thinking of my mum her stories about how she often had rather painful encounters with cows when she was young and had to help on the farm. Bugger! Eventually I mustered the courage to take Ma cow's rope and to pull her aside so I could continue into the jungle. Almost an hour of clambering over a narrow path, over fallen trees, over rocks, over a stream (where is the path now?) but no Tiger Cave to be seen. Instead there were lizards that skittered back into safety, birds that called out, monkeys that were squealing above my head. I did not even dare to think of snakes and other creepy critters. At one point I really didn't know how to proceed. Everywhere I looked I only saw dead ends. So I decided to return. Halfway on my way back I see that a leech had found my big toe and that it was sucking the blood out of it at a rapid pace. I have to say that the way back went much faster than the way there and Ma cow didn't put up any fight, she wisely got out of my way! With the advice of my brother in my head (they let go when in the proximity of fire) I asked for a lighter. "No problem, no problem, water, water" and some hand gestures that I just had to pull it out and keep my foot under water was all I got. EEW! Ever felt a leech before? Now i have, it feels like an earthworm but a bit softer and slimier. Brrr. I still get the creeps when I think of it. I took my sarong and pulled that thing out of my toe with a lot of ooh, ah, eh, ews and cleaned the wound with water. It has bled for a long time after. I stopped at the next beach and examined myself for other of those things. Fortunately there were none. Note to self: If there is only a small chance that you are going in the jungle again, make sure you have decent shoes and long trousers. And take a guide with you! Djees!

Luckily no weird biting animal encounters during the diving trip. Eight meters of depth during 45 minutes. Not bad for a first dive. Honestly, it was awesome! So many fish of all sizes and colors: black, red, blue, orange, striped, speckled, ... Purple starfish, small orange balls that close when you get close. It's impossible to describe it. You have to experience it yourself or watch a documentary on TV. Those schools of fish, changing direction so quickly. Magnificent to see. The colors and shapes of the hard corals. So beautiful. Coming back up I found a bit scary. I wanted to go to the surface as fast as possible, but that is not allowed because of the pressure. You feel the water getting warmer, you see it getting lighter, you can almost taste the air but you still have to stay under water. It was a bit unsettling.

The second dive exceeded the first in all aspects. To start with, there was the pressure in my ears that seemed to bother me much more. It took a little longer to go down because a couple of times I had to go back up a bit to give my ears the time to adjust. But we also went deeper, up to 12 m, so maybe that had something to do with it too. There was so much more to see. Much more life. Not only hard corals but also waving corals. Many more different types of fish, schools of small but also big fish, I even saw a moray eal! Unbelievable! We were down for an hour, it felt like only 5 minutes. But again I felt unsettled on our way to the surface. While I was still recovering from all that beauty, a sudden excitement went through the boat. Dolphins in front of us! Waaaa! Cool! To see them swimming and then suddenly they jump up and do some amazing twists and turns in the air! Breathtaking!

The rhythm of the second week on Koh Lanta was

much slower than that of the first one. Because of the work I'd done with Taro I somehow already knew that you should not take your thoughts so seriously. Yet to apply that in daily life was a real challenge. While outside the thunder and the rain drowned out all the other sounds, I was busy planning the rest of my year. Because oh my god, to not know what would happen in two months. The uncertainty. No way I could handle that. So planning it was. Which countries I wanted to visit? Which months were the best for that? How long would I stay where? Feverishly I searched on the internet, which worked miraculously during those violent storms, for all possible information. While I was planning, I already had a feeling that what I was doing was completely useless. Was it intuition? Call it what you want, something in me told me that you can plan as much as you want, life goes its own way, with or without your plans. I just did not want to believe that voice. In retrospect it was right though. The rest of the year went very differently than I had planned in my innocence. While I was on it, the note with the website of ThaiQiHolistics came back up. Mmm, that seems interesting, let's do those 20 sessions after Indonesia. Let's see if that person really knows that much about energy. Twenty became 2000 (at least) and that person is now my teacher, my Ajahn as they say in Thai, who I respect immensely. But first back to Koh Lanta. Where besides making plans, thoughts had to be examined. As I said above, working with Taro had given me the notion that thoughts should not be taken so seriously. I once borrowed the book by Byron Katie "Loving What Is: Four questions that can change your life" from the library, but I did not understand it, I thought it was all blabla. Taro, however, had told me that it could be an addition to her own teachings. And yes, now it suddenly made sense, now I suddenly understood it. Had the fact that I actually made the assignments in writing this time something to do with it? Probably. It has at least opened my eyes to patterns and it has helped me to step out of those same patterns by questioning my thoughts that lied at the root of them. As Byron Katie herself says so beautifully: "You only suffer when you believe a thought that argues with reality". Most of the time those thoughts contain the word 'should'. I should, I should not, he/she should or should not. Forget should, should is fighting with what is! Forget about fighting, let's go get some fresh air.

Jellyfish, very big jellyfish! I saw them during a walk on the beach. I gladly postponed swimming until the next day. A slightly cuter creature that I encountered during another beach walk was a small lobster, hidden in a shell. And rubbish, a lot of rubbish. Due to low season the beach bars are closed and the beach is no longer cleaned. I was really shocked. The stuff that is washing up on shore! From plastic cups to mattresses! It looks like the ocean has enough of it too. She was as smooth as a mirror last week, this week she is furious. With high roaring foaming waves and strong currents. Everything that we so-called civilized people thrown in her, she spits back out with unrivaled power. All these impressions make hungry. Luckily, my favorite restaurant next to the road stays open all year round. It is always delicious and I love to look in the "kitchen". If you can call it a kitchen. There are two cookers, some bamboo worktables and a number of polystyrene boxes with their fresh produce. But it is so nice to see the lady stirring in her wok, you just see that she does it with love.

I also think back to Koh Lanta with love. Is it because, for the first time, I was really confronted with the fact that thoughts that argue with reality influence your emotions if you allow them? For example, I remember an incredibly beautiful sunset on the beach. I watched with an open mouth and a "waw I am so lucky" feeling. Until the thought: "This would be so much better if my partner had been here now." No less than 2 seconds later the tears ran down my cheeks and I felt miserable. Nothing had changed. The sun was still setting in a mighty colorful spectacle. The only thing that had changed was that I believed a thought that was not real, that was not true. The reality was that that partner was not there. By the way, how could I know if it would have been better? Maybe we would have been arguing at that moment and that fantastic sunset wasn't even noticed. Just to show that thoughts with should are tricksters and you better ignore them. What was real however was that I had to say goodbye to that little island that taught me many valuable insights. It was time to explore Indonesia. When you say Indonesia, you automatically think of Bali. For me, however, Indonesia evokes images of a boat trip through the jungle, orangutans, snorkeling with sea turtles and swimming among jellyfish. Indonesia is so much more than Bali. Yet Bali could not be excluded from our discovery trip through Indonesia.

"Our?"

"Yes, ours." I did not make this trip on my own. Even before I left Belgium, Mariska, a colleague Product Specialist, and I had already made plans to visit Indonesia together. She only had to apply for leave and book her flights. We would meet at the airport. No sooner said than done. Our flights arrived in Jakarta around the same time. We met there and we took another flight to Bali. Bali, oh Bali. That island has something mysterious. It has a certain appeal. After all, we stayed there for 9 days. On the other hand, it has something restless about it. Something that repels me. The hustle and bustle of traffic and being constantly harassed to buy things (taxi miss, car miss, tickets miss, tour miss, ...) certainly contribute to that feeling. Yet I have been back to Bali many times, in very different circumstances. Not to explore the island but to practice Qi Gong for days in a row. I run ahead of myself. First, let's see what Bali had to offer us.

A walk towards Tanjung Benoa. A road straight through the mangrove forest where the locals were fishing on the shore.

... a taxi to Ulu Watu, one of the most important temples of the island. It's a pity that you can not go in. The only thing you can see are aggressive monkeys who grab everything they can get their hands on. That's what people said. Those we have seen behaved more like couch potatoes.

... a refreshing dip, a sunset and a whole plate of goodies, fresh from the sea in Jimbaran. Finger licking good!

... festivities in Ubud. Galungan is a Hindu tradition that is celebrated every 210 days in Bali. The Balinese believe that on that day the spirits of their ancestors descend to earth. To receive them and make them feel welcome they use beautiful decorations and offer huge amounts of food. Along the road are Penjor, long poles decorated with a small altar on which in the morning Balinese ladies wearing their best clothes place small offerings. The same is done in their house temples and in the village temples. And not only the ladies are dressed up, the gentlemen and the children are looking very smart too. After the offerings, the whole family feasts of dishes prepared the day before. Small packets of pork (sacrificial animals) and spicy vegetables in banana leaves. Our hostess gave us too a bunch of these packets. Two types of pork and one with spicy vegetables. Very tasty. I only wonder whether that one type of pork were intestines because it was a bit jelly-like. Maybe it's better not to know.

... a day at the spa and an "extreme bicycle tour". The area around Ubud is very nice to cycle but the organized tours are all similar. They drop you for breakfast in a mega-sized restaurant overlooking the volcano. Afterwards you are taken to a coffee plantation and once you can finally start to cycle it is along the asphalt road and only downhill. We wanted something different. On Internet we found Bayan Tree tours who offered an "extreme bicycle tour" for experienced cyclists along country roads. It was indeed over small roads, sometimes concrete, sometimes not. Between the rice fields, along canals where the women were washing themselves, their children and their clothes. Through the jungle where we spotted monkeys, small komodo dragons and kingfishers. Uphill and downhill, sometimes quite steep, but fun. The guide was full of praise for our cycling. No wonder, the American guy who joined the tour the day before, ended up in one of the canals next to the rice fields!

... a bit of cycling on our own. First towards

the north, then towards the south. Good we did it that way because the north is much more elevated than the south. To get to Tirta Empul, a temple complex built around a bubbling spring, we had to do some serious climbs. Gugung Kawi was only a few hundred meters away from Tirta Empul and there we could see graves or commemorative monuments (they are not sure themselves) of impressive dimensions in a wonderful environment. But before we got to these two monuments we stopped at a local market where we tasted and bought savory tapioca sweets. After lunch, we headed south. Downhill! Fun! Only then I realized how much height difference we covered in the morning. In the South we cycled from one place to another. We looked at a fresco, admired the largest piece of cast metal from the 3rd century BC and sprinkled ourselves with water that would keep us young. After a long day of cycling we ended up at an Italian restaurant for a delicious pizza.

... a tour with a private driver. Via a water palace to Ahmed for snorkeling. Continuing along the winding coastal road high above the sea to finish at the airport.

From Bali it went to Pangkalan Bun for a three day boat trip through the jungle of Indonesian Borneo to spot orangutans. For me that trip could have lasted three days longer. I enjoyed it tremendously. The damp, sticky heat, the mosquitoes, even the dirty, smelly clothes couldn't spoil the fun.

Boarded 'our' klotok early in the morning. Yes, we had a whole boat for us alone. To be honest, that is the normal course of events, but I felt like a queen. It were three amazing days! A culinary boat trip with on the menu three delicious meals per day, the last by candlelight. Again and again the cook conjured up unbelievably tasty food. Add to that the steady rocking of the boat, the hypnotic sound of the engine, beautiful views of the rainforest and lots of monkeys.

We can see these beautiful animals because they are fed in three places. These orangutans were saved from people who kept them as pets. They were reintroduced into the jungle and to ensure that they don't starve they are given extra food. If you are lucky, you will see many at the feeding platforms, if you are unlucky, none. The first orangutans we saw were a mother with her baby and Mum spotted us first. Roaring, she made it clear that she was not so happy with our visit. Luck was with us. We admired another six orangutans around the first feeding platform. Some were very shy, others were real models. The dominant male really liked to be in the spotlight. And from him we had to run away on our way back! He was very near to the path and followed us. Our guide said run, so we ran. A number of other people who did not understand that this is really not a stuffed animal, were pushed out of our way. Safe back in our klotok the captain went looking for a mooring place to spend the night, meanwhile we saw proboscis monkeys and macaques. Then dinner by candlelight with the strumming of a rain shower as background music. Mosquitoes who came feasting along made us turn in early.

The crack of the day and the first sunlight served as our alarm clock. After a full breakfast of toasted bread, scrambled eggs and banana pancake, I took a shower. Meaning: you take a scoop of brown river water from a bucket, you throw it over your head, you soap up and you rinse yourself with another couple of scoops from that same bucket. It gives you a nice soft skin. Ahum. Not that it mattered much because a little later at the second feeding platform I was dripping sweat again. This time the attraction was a squirrel waiting stiffly upside down for his share of the bananas. Fun entertainment until the orangutans arrived. It is undescribable to see them swinging from tree to tree, to observe how there is a hierarchy that is respected: first the male and then the rest. I couldn't get enough of watching them. Also on the third feeding platform it was amazing to observe them. They became quite bold. There was one who waded through the water and pulled the rope with which our boat was tied to a tree. People on other boats were taking pictures but we felt slightly uneasy. After a river water shower and a delicious dinner by candlelight, the stars came out. Stretched out on the deck, looking at thousands of stars and becoming quiet. The third and last day of the orangutan adventure ended with orangutans. And hornbills! Beautiful big mighty birds!

As I reread these words and the memories surface, the more recent images that circulate on the internet also appear. About deforestation and displaced orangutans. Some with burns on their skin due to the policy of slash and burn of the palm oil companies. Entire parts of the jungle are burned down to plant palm trees. To satisfy the demand from the West for cheap palm oil that you can find in almost all chocolate spreads and biscuits. Large parts of the jungle that we visited then, have already disappeared together with their inhabitants. Residents who wouldn't hurt a fly, beautiful creatures of mother nature who like us just want to live. It makes me sad to know that my godchild, and not only him, will probably not be able to enjoy this beauty anymore. Let us hope that I'm wrong and that in fifteen or twenty years I can make the same trip again with him. And who knows, we can also go to Yogyakarta to see two world-famous monuments, Prambanan and Borobudur. I suppose there is much less chance that they will have disappeared. Especially Borobudur I found to be very impressive. Yet Angkor Wat, until now, for me, is the temple encountered on my travels in Asia that appeals the most to one's imagination. Even the Temple of Heaven in Beijing, beautiful in its own way, cannot match Angkor Wat. But back to Prambanan and Borobudur. Especially the way to the latter was not paved with roses.

A round Yogyakarta we find two famous monuments. One even features on the cover of the Lonely Planet of Indonesia. Day 1 brought us to Prambanan early in the morning. Six large Hindu temples in close proximity. They are dedicated to the three major Hindu gods and their respective mounts. The biggest and the most interesting one, dedicated to Shiva was in renovation and unfortunately forbidden to enter.

From Prambanan to Borobudur. Three buses, three hours and a lot of annoyances later we arrived at the hotel. Annoyances? Well, yes. To change buses, we had to wait at a closed-off bus stop, stacked like sardines in a tin. When the right bus arrived, we were, very subtle (not!), pushed to the side so there was no chance we would get on that bus. When we finally managed to get on the third bus for Borobudur, with at least 15 people and 3 chickens too many, someone found it a good idea to start smoking. Add sticky bodies, the lovely odors of fresh and not so fresh sweat and a bus that could disintegrate at any moment and you'll get the picture.

The same night we got up at 4am and jumped on the back of a motorcycle to Setumbu Hill to see the sunrise over the Buddhist temple of Borobudur. It was worth the trouble. You saw it getting lighter, all shades of pink appeared, fog rose from the forest and formed clouds (Oh no, there goes our sunrise!) and then suddenly a bright red disc appeared between the two hills. After conquering her first shyness, she ascended to heaven faster and faster. Beautiful! From the Hill it went to the temple which was still completely covered in fog when we arrived. The monument itself was much more impressive than that of Prambanan. 123 m in square and 32 m high. Fully covered with bas-reliefs depicting the life of Buddha and 300 seated Buddha statues. You can easily spend half a day there but our motorcycle guides told us that two hours was sufficient. They wanted to show us two other smaller temples, so after two hours we said goodbye to Borobudur. Next to the last temple there was a large tree with lianas that looked very inviting. We couldn't resist playing the monkey. Now we know how Tarzan feels. After a late breakfast of nasi goreng, the view of the rice field from our balcony was the background of some deep philosophical discussions.

Philosophical discussions, you know. About Life and stuff, about men and stuff, and some more about men, you know. From philosophical musings to volcano climbing is only a small step. Especially if you have to get up at 4 o'clock in the morning.

I can assure you that it was painful to hear the alarm! The Merapi is the world's most active volcano which is astounding because you do not see lava, you do not hear any sounds and you do not feel heat. You only see a plume of smoke coming out of the top. But it has taken people's lives during the eruptions in 2006 and 2010. In 2010, Yogyakarta, which is 42 km away, was covered with a 10 cm layer of ashes! We took a hike through newly grown forest where you could still see the evidence of the devastating power of the volcano. In some parts we had to climb on hands and feet over fallen tree trunks. After two and a half hours through forest, elephant grass and dry riverbeds we arrived on what they call the lava plain. The bunker where two journalists who felt safe were killed, roasted by ash clouds of more than 1500°C, got me the creeps. We were at that moment in the dangerous zone. It's forbidden for tourists. Only with special permission and a guide you can go there. If the volcano would erupt, much chance you wouldn't make it. But there are 7 observation posts and the guide was in contact with them via walkie talkie. In the case of strongly increased activity, we would be warned and would have to leave the area immediately together with the residents. After a trip of six hours in total I was happy with the extensive breakfast that was waiting for us. The bus ride back to Yogyakarta was one of extremes. The first 45 minutes went by at a speed of 10 km an hour, then the driver got a phone call and started racing and doing crazy maneuvers. I guess he suddenly had to be home for dinner. Anyway, I was glad to get out of that bus. My ankles not so much. They went on strike. You should have seen me. A crooked old ladie would have walked much faster than me.

Since I discovered Qi Gong, my ankles have never hurt that badly anymore. You can ask Mariska, two days later I was still limping. And biting my teeth against the pain. I was about to cry, it could not go on like this, could it? I cursed my youthful self and her stupidity. The pains started when, around the age of thirteen, I had a tear in the ligaments of my right ankle. I vehemently refused a cast, I went through that on my tenth because of a fracture in the right elbow. A supportive tape was all I allowed the doctor to put on. Three weeks later I was already performing during a gymnastics interclub competition. Ah yes, young and stupid. It has cost me more than 20 years of pain. A night out and dancing equaled rolling out of my bed the next morning like an 80 year old. A day of shopping? Idem. Yoga did not bring any improvement. Qi Gong did. How? Well, Qi Gong looks at your alignment. Physically and energetically. First, a lot of physical adjustments have to be made and they are all based on posture. In the exercises you will learn a different, more aligned, relaxed posture that slowly will seep into your daily life. That's the first step which already brings huge improvements. Besides less ankle pain my x-shaped legs disappeared. Second, things must be released. Your posture can be perfect, if you hold it, and it being your energy, the pain will come back. Even now, after more than 4 years and 5000 hours of Qi Gong practice, there are times when I hold it. With pain as a result. The moment I can let go, in the correct alignment, do not ask me how, I can not answer that, the pain disappears like snow in the sun. And the sun brings us back to Indonesia where the last days were spent on an idyllic island. Or was that just appearances?

During the ride I was shocked by the deforestation that is happening on Indonesian Borneo. Everywhere you look, you see parts of burnt down forest where only a few lonely tree stumps are still standing while smoke is lingering around the black ashes of a once green lush jungle. Above it a magnificent sunset. Surreal! We got to Derawan, our paradise island for the last few days. Paradise, however, was somewhat disappointing. Many hostels were fully booked, the rooms that were free were dirty and the prices were skyhigh. With no ATM's on the island we had stocked up based on prices mentioned in a travel guide with some extra margin but the prices they asked us were double or triple. What?! So we took the first room that was a bit reasonably priced and where there was no mold on the walls.

Fortunately we could move to a bungalow on the water after two nights in a slightly less pleasant room. The last night however, we spent in a homestay. More about that later. From the terrace of our bungalow we were able to admire many beautiful creatures. To begin with, sea turtles who came to graze in front of your door. I took the snorkel, jumped into the water and went swimming with them. It was a race. They won! So fast that they are! You wouldn't say when you look at them from above but try to keep up with them when you're in the water. Even with flippers you lose. They came every day around the same hour to get their grass meal. If you went snorkeling guaranteed you could see them. The highlight for me was seeing 5 of those giant animals together.

The stingray I admired from afar. I didn't want to end up like Crocodile Dundee. He died because he was stung by one. I was not too keen on the sea snake either. The starfish was the one that made us stare in the water for an hour. We saw a moray eel, the sea snake mentioned above, a puffer fish, trumpet fish, a butterfly-like fish and some others. We were lucky, there was no wind and the water was crystal clear.

The second night on the island we were sitting on the beach to look at the stars. Suddenly, a black form appears from the water. Looking closer, it turned out that it was a turtle who, after making a tour, had found the right place to dig a hole and lay her eggs. Nice to see, too bad that at the end of the process a bunch of locals arrived with a lot of noise and LED lights from their cell phones. Poor turtle mum... A day or two later I released three little tortoises back in the sea. When we returned from our dinner, I had a chat with a local while Mariska was playing ping pong with the local youth. Suddenly the gentleman told me that he had tortoises and that he was going to release them. Did I wanted to help? Sure! At first it seemed like they wanted to go back to the tub from which they came but after taking a turn they were on their way. Safe journey, little ones!

The underwater world in and around Derawan is really amazing. The corals that grow on the pillars of the bungalows and attract enormous schools of fish are beautiful to see. It is a pity that there is a lot of waste floating in the water around the island. And it has a negative influence. Closer to the coast, many corals have already died. When I spoke to an Indonesian man who threw his empty packet of cigarettes into the water, he started to give up on the government. That it was their fault. They had stopped garbage collection. Could be but it is not the government that throws waste into the water, it is the people who do that. Twice we were able to escape to other (still) idyllic islands. Both times we joined a 3-islands tour so the price would be affordable for all participants.

Apart from snorkeling near each of the islands, we swam on Kakaban between the jellyfish. They don't sting anymore because they are in a closed salt water lake where they have no enemies. I must admit that it's a very strange feeling, jellyfish that bump into you. At first I gave a few shrieks through my

snorkel but afterwards it was more giggling.
And now about the homestay. The bottom
line is that you just sleep in a room in
people's homes. We found one at a very
reasonable price, the bathroom was somewhat clean and the hostess spoke a little bit
of English. She served us tea in the evening and breakfast twice in the morning. Yes
really. First the sweet doughnut-like things
with tea. An hour later she tells us that
breakfast is ready. Huh? Didn't we just had
breakfast? Turned out she had prepared four
(!) fish. Two grilled and two fried, with rice
and a spicy lime sauce. To eat sitting on the
floor. A great meal and the best spicy sauce
that I have eaten during our time in Indonesia. It complemented perfectly with the
fish. When we had finished eating, it was
their turn to eat, also fish with rice and also
on the floor. She then arranged our transport
back to Kalimantan. Came in handy ... and
I didn't mind the extra rupees that we paid
too much for it.

And with that the Indonesian adventure ended and
the Qi Gong adventure was about to start.

PART II

The discovery of Qigong

About the first steps

(June 2014- Feb 2015)

5. QI GONG:
THE BEGINNING

Four flights and two days later I am back in Thailand. In Chiang Mai. To start a 20-day Qi Gong course. Something totally new for me.

Who would have thought that those 20 days would turn out to be more than 3 years? My Qi Gong adventure started June 17, 2014 and still goes on today. That first day started off really well. Right. When I parked my bicycle, I bumped into the hot exhaust pipe of a motorcycle with my calf. Damn that was painful! Guaranteed I left some pieces of skin behind there. After the wound was taken care of, I had my first conversation with Ajahn. There would be many more to come but that first conversation was rather special. He asked me why I was there for. A bit taken aback I answered:

"Uhm, during yoga I started to feel energy and I wanted to know more about that. Someone who has followed a course with you told me that you know a lot about energy. "

He smiled a bit, didn't really answer, but asked me if I

had any physical problems.

"Uhm, not really no. Well, yes, my ankles hurt after a long walk. And I have lordosis, but that's already from childhood, nothing to do about that. In any case, the abdominal exercises from the physiotherapist have not helped. "

He looks at me with what I came to call his Qi Gong X-ray eyes and says: "We can do something about those ankles, your back will improve and your toes will get straight too." "Hmm" was all I had to say all the while thinking: "Yeah, right!". Just to indicate that I was very skeptical. He avoided my questions about energy and the things I was not really into, my toes for God's sake, he thought important. It would all become clear to me later. Not much later because already after 6 classes I knew that I would stay a little longer in Chiang Mai. To be honest, I knew it already after the second class, but my skeptic self didn't want to accept it yet.

Please do not take the impressions of those first sessions too literally. I speak a lot about energy because that was what I deemed important, which I wanted to concentrate on. In reality, it's not about that at all. The energy is something that comes from the right posture, from letting go and from being in center. Controlling, sending etc is all blahblah, a story that my mind told about the reality of not being in center. I know now that in the TQH way of teaching, which I also follow, the teachings are adapted to the moment and to the condition of your body but always with finding your center in mind. Since your body is different every time, every day, the guidelines can also be different. If you lean too far back on day 1 I will say that you have to come forward, if you lean too much forward on day 2 then I will say that you have to come back. The intention is to find your center. And this is how I experienced it back then.

T he main thing I am in Chiang Mai for is to learn Qi Gong. Qi what? Qi Gong. Pronounced as "Chee Gung". Qi Gong is a traditional Chinese health system. Qi is the life force or energy that is present in all things and Gong is skill. Qi Gong literally means the ability to deal with life energy. It is a system that is used to maintain health, increase vitality and promote healing. Qi Gong uses physical postures, breathing techniques and focused concentration. There are different Qi Gong styles that range from the soft internal (yin) styles such as Tai Chi to external, powerful (yang) styles such as Kung Fu. However, the slow and smooth movements of most Qi Gong forms can easily be adapted to every body and can be practiced by all age groups.

So far for the theory. The practice goes as follows. I do these exercises every day in the morning from 10 to 13h and fall asleep every afternoon on my bed for two hours! Honestly! For the first time on Tuesday I cycled to the clinic where I met Ajahn Toh, my teacher. The clinic has three treatment rooms where Ajahn treats patients with acupuncture, Qi Massage and Qi Gong. In the corridor that connects the rooms, I do, together with two or three other students, my exercises. Ajahn is Indonesian of Chinese descent and learned his art from several masters. He told me the first day that in this month I would learn the 7 statics (7 standing exercises) which would improve my posture, the arched back less arched and the flat feet less flat, in addition he would give me some acupuncture to open my ankles so that I am no longer an old lady after a walk of 6 hours and also the acne he could cure. Meanwhile I got all 7 exercises on 4 days. Now it is a matter of perfecting them. To do them from my Dantian (the area just below the navel). Ajahn thinks I have a lot of control over my body, I progress very fast and I can understand him when he talks about connection with the Dantian. That is why I am allowed to do some less static exercises. Exercises that remind me of my year of Kung Fu: forward kicks and back and forth steps. The forward kicking-stepping goes as follows: find your stance, find your Dantian, kick from your Dantian, balance, feel the connection with your toes, come back to your center, then put your foot down, with control, heel first, then your toes and put that foot straight, do not let the knee fall in and watch your breathing. You wobble because you hold your energy too high, let it sink to your Dantian. Uhuh, okay. I find it easier to step backwards because it reminds me of tango.

I have now practiced the 7 statics for six days and I notice that I am already standing differently on my feet. My ankles actually fall less inwards. My body adapts, probably that's the reason why I need an afternoon nap every day in addition to my normal 9 hours of sleep! I think I arrived in Chiang Mai at the right time. Because of the rainy season many of Ajahn's students are back home. Those who are staying are those who follow an instructor training and have been in Chiang Mai for more than a year. Which is great because I train with them and get the same information. I also get a lot more individual coaching because we are so few. Lovely! My first acupuncture session is also a fact. My right foot looked like a pincushion. It was not painful, but I felt strange sensations in my groin. Yes, I find it interesting here, I even feel like I'm going to stay a little longer than the foreseen month. But let's see. For now I don't do much more than cycling to the clinic for half an hour, three hours of training, cycling back, looking for food, taking an afternoon nap, a bit of swimming, enjoying the sun, a bit of reading and a bit of meditation. No explorations of Chiang Mai yet, I didn't even go for a massage. The energy is lacking. The only thing I did do was buying new t-shirts on the Saturday Walking Street, a big market for which they completely shut down one of the busiest streets of Chiang Mai for all traffic. My white t-shirts worn in the jungle were no longer white. I happily replaced them with more colorful ones.

Together with the purchase of those colorful t-shirts, the yoga era was left behind. If I remember correctly, I did headstand only twice during the first Qi Gong week and that was it. Firstly, the effect that Qi Gong had on my energy level was profound and secondly, I began to understand that in Qi Gong the way of moving and dealing with your body is so much softer. No painful stretches, no impossible twisted postures, no strange breathing and abdominal rotation techniques. And certainly not standing on your head! Just, simple standing or sitting exercises. Which doesn't mean that they are easy! I wanted more!

I've decided, I will stay a whole lot longer in Chiang Mai than I had first planned. What I have seen and felt this week has convinced me. It is unbelievable how my body responds to Qi Gong and acupuncture. On Monday, Wednesday and Friday I underwent acupuncture sessions in the afternoon in addition to the normal Qi Gong practice in the morning. No more afternoon naps. But the strange thing was that I actually didn't need them anymore. In contrast to the first needle session of Sunday, extra wires were used on Monday and Wednesday. Electricity was put on the needles via mini booster cables. A very strange feeling and at times a bit painful, especially in the beginning when they have to turn the buttons to get the voltage right. Sometimes there is no need for electricity, that needle between my thumb and forefinger. Djeez, what was that?! That aaaawww came from my toes! Needles in my stomach, in my lower legs, in my feet and in my ankles. Wires on my stomach, legs and feet. It felt like I was participating in some weird science experiment. Yet there was a system behind that experiment. The needles were mainly on the stomach meridian. What does that have to do with a painful ankle you ask? Apparently I have energy stagnation in the stomach area which would explain my belly (I carry all that energy in front) and my arched back (no energy there, only open space). By carrying the energy in front, my body posture is not completely straight and my center of gravity is more at the front of my feet and ankles than nicely in the middle. My old ankle injury therefore plays up. But now something can be done about it. The energy that is stuck can be loosened and my body can be re-balanced. Both can be done with the Qi Gong exercises but acupuncture, or Qi-massage for the matter, accelerates the process. You bet! My belly has been bloated and tight all week and I look as if I am 6 months pregnant. According to Ajahn (which is the Thai word for teacher), it's only temporary. Let us hope it is! According to him, I have to direct the energy released by the acupuncture to my feet, clearly I can't manage that yet. But there is progress. The arch in my back, which has been needled on Friday, seems to have diminished. My ankle is protesting when I stand 'normally'. When I stand with my weight in the middle of my feet, the protesting stops. For me, however, it feels like I'm going to fall backwards. That feeling diminishes when I tilt my hips forward which in turn makes me feel like I'm a collapsed pudding. When I look in the mirror, I 'm actually pretty straight! How your brain can deceive you!

Every morning I practice the 7 statics and try to apply the above mentioned concepts. Apparently I do it quite okay because I now also have to apply them in a flowing form called the '7 star form'. Normally it's not something that you are taught during your first month of practice, but Ajahn thinks that I will develop faster, that my body will re-align faster by applying the concepts in motion. But that is only possible if you have enough body awareness. And according to him, I have that because of my gymnastics, rope skipping, kung fu and karate background. I agree. If he says put your feet parallel, they are parallel, knee above the ankle is knee above the ankle. Only when the heel has to be placed first my body has its own will. I can think all I want: "heel first", seven times out of ten my toes are first on the floor. Remains of the drill during gymnastics.

You may have noticed that I am not yet talking about energy and controlling and sending energy. I am absolutely not there yet. For now, the focus is only on the physical aspect. The energy comes later when the body is properly aligned. What I do feel sometimes is a kind of heat, but in the wrong place. In my ears. If you've ever been pulled by your ears you know what I mean. That warm, throbbing feeling. That is what I feel in the second static exercise (without being pulled by my ears!) I should feel it in my fingertips. Forget about sending it, I still keep it in my shoulders. Yes, I feel that, in my ears. Ugh.

A second aspect that has played a role in the decision to further dive into the Qi Gong practice is that I think there is much more wisdom to find in Qi Gong than in yoga. As far as I can assess and compare after only two weeks, I can say the following: I did yoga for two years and my ankles didn't change, the pain of the old injury remained. Two weeks into Qi Gong and a lot has changed. Yoga works, just like Qi Gong, with energy but in a very different way. According to Ajahn with imagination and I have to agree with him. In yoga it was so often repeated how the energy flows that you will eventually start to feel it. In Qi Gong Ajahn didn't tell me anything about energy flows, he didn't even want to answer when I asked those questions. He said that with practice I would experience that for myself and then it would be real, not from a kind of indoctrination. When I said that my ears were getting warm, he laughed: "Real energy, no imagination but wrong place, send it to your fingers." I have to figure out how to do that myself. It's called a challenge. Another difference between yoga and Qi Gong is the use of energy. Yoga uses it to reach enlightenment as quickly as possible, Qi Gong uses it to heal your body and help other people heal theirs. They use the Buddhist/Taoist doctrine to go deeper into spirituality. What this system, and I mean the system applied by Ajahn, makes it even more interesting for me is his way of combining his knowledge of acupuncture, massage, Chinese medicine, Thai medicine, Ayurveda, Western medicine and spirituality into an individual approach for each of his patients and his instructors. I could not put my finger on it on day 2, when I already had the feeling that I would stay here for a while, but it's that combination that has done it.

The third aspect of the decision to stay was what I saw happening with a crippled man. Imagine a huge guy, 1m90, 120 kg who wears a brace on both feet, tilts to his right side, walks with a walking stick and has to be supported by two other huge guys not to fall over because he is limping so much. That is how I saw him coming into the clinic for the first time, about a week and a half ago. My first thought was that he must have had a serious accident. Later it turned out that he had five bullets in his back, some of which could not be removed. Too dangerous. The reason of the bullets I don't know. In the meantime he's been in the clinic 5 or 6 times. He receives Qi Gong exercises based on the 7 statics, which he does sitting on a stool and which are adapted to his condition. After he has spent about an hour doing this, he gets an acupuncture treatment. It is incredible to see what progress that man has made! He now walks with a walker and does not have to be supported anymore. The first time with the walker he was still tilting to one side and the walker had to be moved and held by his helpers. Now he does everything by himself and he is not leaning over to one side anymore. And that after one and a half week! This, along with the changes in my own body, has made me realize what a powerful system this is. One in which I want to immerse myself much deeper, hence the decision to spend the rest of my sabbatical year in Thailand.

Yes but what about traveling? And all those beautiful things that you are not going to see now? Those beautiful things do not run away, I can visit them during other holidays that will come. I only have one chance to immerse myself in a life-changing system for 6 months. So I want to grab that opportunity while I have the chance. Maybe I should change the name of my blog because yoga is no longer involved. This week has flown by! I like it here.

The next 2 weeks also flew by. There were so many things to learn, to experience and to describe. Which does not mean that I did not suffer and that no emotions were involved. But something deep inside me knew that this time it was worth it. And so I kept on going and I tried to give it a place for myself by writing it down in detail on the blog.

I will start with the physical symptoms. The swollen belly has disappeared. It is not yet flat but maybe the delicious Thai food has something to do with that. The curve in my back has really reduced. I'm not imagining this! When I was in bed yesterday, I felt that I was more supported than usual. To be certain that it was not the mattress, I stretched out on the floor. It was the first time in my life that I could not slide a hand between my lower back and the floor. Whoo-haaa !!! My ankle has passed the ultimate test: walking around on Saturday Walking Street at a super-slow pace for three hours because there were so many people that I could not go any faster. And on flip flops. Previously guaranteed I would have problems the next day. Now, nothing! My ankle only hurts when I don't stand correctly. That is, with my weight not in the middle of my feet or my feet not nicely parallel. The collapsed pudding feeling gradually disappeared. Now, if I stand like I always used to stand, it feels unnatural.

And what about the energy? It's getting there, slowly. I do not feel any heat in my ears anymore but that does not mean that I can send it to my fingertips. I still keep it partly in my shoulders, at the point where your arms start. And to make me more aware of it, Ajahn has put a needle there on both sides. With those needles in my shoulders and one under my navel I had to stand in front of the mirror and do the first static exercise. Just a matter of making the connection between these three points. Yeah, easier said than done!

For the skeptics who do not believe in energy at all, I have two anecdotes which knocked me off my socks. But first I have to tell you about a young man of 29 who torn the ligaments of his ankle due to a wrong step. There has been an operation to restore them by using metal pins. One morning during his recovery he suddenly could no longer lift his foot. It's called drop foot. We have been in class together three times this week. And because it is better for him not to stand too long on his foot, we did all exercises sitting on a stool. They are the same "simple" exercises that I normally do standing up. By doing them sitting, I learned a lot, I understand better now what is meant by "connecting" and then the energy aspect emerges.

And that's where my first anecdote fits in. At one point I was totally frustrated. After hearing about 100 times that I lost the connection, that I held it with my muscles and that I had to let it go to my fingers, I cried out: "But what do you mean by that, I don't understand!" Ajahn has shown me. In two ways.

Keep in mind that he is a skinny, wiry man.

He stands in the posture (make fists, bring them at the height of your chest towards each other so that you form a kind of circle but your knuckles don't touch) and says: "Push my forearms inwards"

I push...

No movement.

He says: "Harder".

I push with my full weight as hard as I can.

I can't get his arms moving.

Huh?

I can not even push a skinny, wiry man his arms inwards?

He says, with a laugh in his voice for my wonderment: "That was connection, there is energy between my arms." "And now I'm going to do the same but with my muscles, push again."

I push again, I feel the resistance of the muscles but they give in and with some effort I can push his arms inwards.

"That's what you do, please stand."

I get into the posture. He pushes on my shoulders and says "connection okay", he pushes on my elbows and says, "Connection okay, you feel that, I can not push them in." He pushes on my forearms and they immediately give in. It's clear, no connection there. What I remember most is not that I did not have a connection in my forearms but that I did have it in my elbows. And especially the feeling when he tried to push them towards each other. They did not budge and I did not have to make any effort for that! Amazing!

Anecdote two: And this really blew me away! The crippled man came, just like the two previous weeks, three times for his treatment. On one of those days we did the sitting exercises together. One is to make a kind of rocking motion in which you bring your knee up and then put your foot firmly back on the floor. Of course you have to make the connection between your toes of the foot that's lifted and your DanTian (your center under your navel). After doing this a number of times with the right foot, the foot in which this guy has no feeling anymore, Ajahn suddenly says: "Yes, this is what you need, you see" and he starts kicking against that foot. And I mean, really kicking. That foot does not move a millimeter! "That's what Qi is, that's what Qi does, you see!" Half a minute later he gives it a small flick with his hand and the foot flies about 20 cm sideways. "But for you it is only temporary, keep on practicing" is his laconic comment. I think my eyes almost popped out of my head!

Next to Qi Gong I gained a lot of other knowledge this week. Among other Buddhist meditation methods to be and stay more concentrated and which for me are very valuable but with which I do not want to bore you. It would lead me too far to explain terms such as samadhi, sati, panya, vittaka and vicara. Those who are interested should come to class one time. Also very interesting is the basis of Chinese medicine: the yin/yang principle and the 5 elements and how this affects our organs. Which organs are yin, which are yang, which element connects to which organ and what does that mean? Fascinating! And this was just the beginning. The explanation about the meridians is still to come. Do you now understand why I want to stay here for another 6 months? This is so extensive and so different from what I know from all my previous studies! And although I want to go deeper into the theory, it is the practice that really keeps me here. Can I learn to play with my energy, with my Qi? And can I influence my health, my body? So far it turns out to be a very clear yes. I do the same exercises a hundred times, perhaps a thousand times, and yet they are always different. Every time I do them, another part of the puzzle is revealed. And I begin to see and feel cohesion. Let's continue with the puzzle image, shall we? I think everyone has ever made a puzzle. You start by spreading out all the pieces, the drawing facing up. Then you find the edge pieces and try to fit them together. Then you finish the inside. Usually there is not much logic in the latter. You have some pieces that fit together here, the same over there and also a small part somewhere else. It's only a matter of time and patience to put of all those small pieces together into one big picture. That's what I'm doing now, puzzling. I'm just at the beginning of my puzzle. I am spreading the pieces and fitting the edge pieces together. And because I do 7 statics and 7 star (7 static exercises and 20 fluid exercises) you can say that I'm making 27 puzzles at the same time. Which are then linked to each other again. A kind of 3D puzzle. The edge of some exercises has been formed and the inside is starting to become clearer. On some I can't even put the edge together. Exercise three is one of them. I can not get a grip on it, it drives me crazy.

In my moments of frustration Ajahn shares his wisdom. Here are some of his expressions. My reaction to it, out loud or not, I have added for the sake of completeness.

"You think too much! You have already a PhD with your mind, now get one with your body! "

-> AAARGH, I know! I haven't found the off button yet. If you know where to find it, please tell me!

"I give you one thing and you lose it all. Too much awareness there. "

-> huh? I did not know that you could have

too much awareness. But it is true, if I focus too much on one thing, the rest, which normally goes well, starts to go off. Interesting!

"It's only illusion, my leg does not move."

-> no? Seems to me it's moving. Can you do that again? Ah yes, interesting, it does stay in the same position. And how do you do that? From your center? Ah okay.

"Aaah, you see, now you understand it, eh! It's as simple as 1 + 1 = 2 "

-> big smile. Yes, I feel the difference. But how is he seeing that there is connection or not? For me it looks exactly the same.

That last statement made me smile. Seeing connection in others is something that you learn by finding the connection in your own body. It is something that requires practice and time. It comes when it comes. You can not force it. You may be able to lend a hand by observing the posture of your fellow students and looking at the effect of the corrections on their alignment in addition to your own practice. Not for beginners, this! As a beginner you wrestle with other things. Like flow and settle at the same time.

"Flow! ... But settle first ... Don't stop! Settle ... and flow!"

How to explain this? The bottom line is that the motions have to be flowing, that I can not stop, but that I still have to find a place to rest in the movements. I struggled a whole morning to finally give up trying to understand it. And then suddenly it clicked. Letting go was the key.

In the meantime, my increased need for sleep has reappeared. Tuesday afternoon (after a night of 11 hours of sleep!) and Friday and Saturday afternoon an afternoon nap was needed. Strong stuff, this Qi Gong thing. No acupuncture this week. Apparently Qi Gong exercises are all my body need to adjust. And it is adjusting, I can feel that. Suddenly a stabbing pain in my shoulder joint. You know, there where I hold the energy, although I never realized that myself. Because pain is nothing more and nothing less than a signal to adjust your posture so that the energy can flow again (another statement from Ajahn) I tried to do that. No luck, it did not help. So I called him to find the right posture which turned out not to be easy. "Relax, relax!" Yeah but how do you do that when it hurts?

Good question! And one that I have never found and probably never will find an unambiguous answer to. Qi Gong works with the whole, it works with body and mind. Is the pain purely caused by the body? Or is there a mental component involved? Up to the student to find out for himself. As an instructor you can only say "Relax." Which I find very difficult. I would love to say to students in pain what they have to do to get rid of the pain. But from my own experience I know that it doesn't work that way. Sometimes is does but when your posture, your alignment is correct, the only thing I can give you is "relax". This student, however, did not find that sufficient and wanted a little more explanation.

I asked Ajahn after the class why I never had problems with my shoulders until the yoga TTC and now again during Qi Gong. Why is it that I have pain with movement and not in daily life? The answer was that in daily life the body is so used to that wrong posture (raised shoulders) that it will consider it 'good'. By doing yoga and Qi Gong you 'force' your body in other positions where it has to let go of that wrong posture. As a result, it suddenly realizes that there is a different way of doing things. The body now feels the difference between wrong and blocked and good and flowing, first during exercise, later also in daily life. From the moment it is now blocked, it gives a pain signal. To let you know: "Hey, something's wrong here, do something about it!" I had to consider it a good thing. It meant that I could relax more in the postures, that I use my muscles less and therefore cut off the energy less.

What have we learned? That I think too

much, that I have to let go and that muscles
are not always an advantage ...

I have experienced many times that muscles are not
always an advantage. In fact, you can safely say that
they are never an advantage. They are needed to
move your body but that's it. You do not have to train
them. You certainly do not have to strengthen them.
The only thing you achieve is that they cut off your
Qi. And it's your Qi that takes care of your strength
and your health. You don't want to cut that off, do
you? I speak from experience when I say that it takes
a very long time to undo the effects of muscle training. Even now, almost 5 years later, there are muscles
in my body that I sometimes unconsciously tense. My
biceps, for instance. I can assure you that that is not
a nice feeling and if it goes on long enough, all sorts
of other problems arise. Problems that you would rather want to avoid and which are actually easy to
prevent: "Relax those biceps Ils!" To do that, I had to
make sure that I could continue practicing.

6. INSTRUCTOR COURSE: THE FIRST 6 MONTHS.

In order to continue to focus on Qi Gong, I first had to make sure that I could stay in Thailand. Without a visa you can stay in the country for a month and that month was over for me. I had to leave the country irrevocably. At that time you could still go to Laos for a double entry visa that, if you planned it well, gave you the right to stay for 6 months in Thailand, with a border run after 3 months. Nowadays that is no longer the case. I made a virtue of necessity and visited the usual tourist attractions in and around Luang Prabang while I waited for my visa. Qi Gong was not put on hold. There was homework to be done.

Homework? Yes, Ajahn told me to do my Qi Gong exercises (the 7 static and the 7 star) every day. I amaze myself by actually doing them every day. I'm normally not that good at that kind of stuff. Or I do not feel like it, or I have something else to do, or ... You know them those excuses. But no, not this time. It must be that Qi Gong has something more than all the rest I've been working on so far. And sweating that I am when I'm practicing. The air conditioning at 21 degrees and still I'm dripping. Odd, because when you watch it as an outsider you see a girl standing still while waving a bit with her arms. Another part of the homework is to translate my blog posts from the previous month in English so that Ajahn can read them. Quite the job, but one more post to go and then I am done. It feels strangely vulnerable, it's like I'm back in high school and have to hand in my essay. No good memories there. My Dutch language teacher once told me that I wasn't able to write a decent piece of text.

That teacher is probably right, I will never win the Pulitzer prize. As long as my teaching talent exceeds my writing talent, I'm not complaining. And now we are back at Qi Gong. There was a decision to make, whether or not to start the Instructor Training. I had already said no twice to Ajahn because I felt that, the wise words at the end of the yoga training in mind, I practiced Qi Gong for myself, not to teach and I didn't see the added benefits of yet another certificate. Now, Ajahn is not someone who distributes certificates, he is not doing that at all and the trajectory of this kind of Qi Gong doesn't lend itself to that. It is not one-size-fits-all. Although we are all doing the same exercises, everyone reacts in his or her own way. Physically, mentally and spiritually. You cannot just say: "Okay, you have completed 500 hours of Qi Gong class, you can now start to teach." That's not the way this system works. When Ajahn proposed it a third time, I asked him why it was so important to do this Instructor Training. The answer may have been a bit more complicated than how I describe it here but it comes down to the fact that if you do the Instructor Training you commit yourself, also financially, to do 100 sessions. This gives Ajahn a long-term vision for you. If you only commit for 20 sessions, he only has a vision for those 20 sessions. Because I had chosen to stay for 6 months anyway, it would be better for me as well as for Ajahn to do the Instructor Course. I let it sink in for a couple of days and I finally decided to give it a go. Not with teaching as a goal, but to get to know my body and my Qi. Which sometimes went well, sometimes less well. And sometimes it led to hilarious situations. A selection from the varied range, more or less in chronological order.

We got a new student in class. Her energy is rather, how shall I say it? Like everywhere and no-where. She can not focus for longer than 2 minutes, is distracted by the least, has no body awareness and doesn't accept corrections very well. For some reason she always ends up next to me. It seems that Ajahn is doing that on purpose, putting her between me and Seijin because we are apparently well-focused and well-grounded. He thinks this is an ideal learning experience for us. And I thought I would ask if I could take a little more distance because I felt distracted by her. I guess I'll have to learn to deal with it and find a balance between concentration and distraction.

That balance didn't come easy.

Especially in the beginning it was as if I took over all her weird body positions. Nothing seemed to work, I was frustrated and then off course it didn't work at all anymore. After a few deep in- and exhalations, I had found my 'focused and well-grounded' self again and things improved. Strange how someone can have such an influence. I am already glad that my fellow students felt it too.

About massage:

What a lucky girl I am! Getting a foot massage and the other time a full body massage for free. Ajahn had decided that my fellow students had to practice their Qi Massage and because I haven't followed that course yet, I had to lend my body to science and undergo the experiment. I felt so bad about that (definitely not!). Let me explain what Qi Massage entails. It is a massage technique that uses the acupuncture points and exercises pressure on them but much less than eg a Thai massage. The pressure is usually maintained longer and gradually increased. In addition, the masseur/masseuse uses his/her own energy to let the energy flow into the "patient". You can really feel that. Not only by the warmth of the hands of the person who gives the massage but also by the tingling in your own body. I was assigned to Luis. She had massaged me at the beginning of my Qi Gong adventure, just before one of my acupuncture sessions, and said that she felt a difference, that I was better aligned, that she did not have to stop my feet going the wrong way anymore. Nice to hear from someone else that positive change is really happening.

Some months later, there was other good news:

I have been again the subject of Qi Massage. Always nice to get a free massage and especially if there are three pairs of hands working with you ... Apparently it was meant to show how to relax a hollow back but I must have kind of ruined it. Ajahn calls me after class and says he was surprised that my back was so relaxed. He said he had to improvise because there was in fact nothing more to relax. "Okay, that's great news but how come I still have the lordosis?" He answered that it is because I cannot relax my thighs yet.

These thighs were not only the cause of my lower back problems, they also had an influence on something else which I only found out later.

According to Ajahn, I'm making progress. There are small changes that he finds very important. Like the sides of my feet. Who could have thought that they would prove important? Of all the body parts a man can look at, he picks the sides of my feet. Well anyway: most people I know can stand on the outsides of their feet. I can not. Never could. No matter how much effort I put in, my feet stay flat on the ground, they refuse to turn open. I thought that had to do with my flat feet but here they have a different theory about it. It seems that I always tense my thighs without realizing it myself. It's such a natural state for me that I don't even feel it. And therefore, those feet do not open. And now suddenly they did! Not completely off course but the inside came a bit off the ground. Which means that I start to relax my thighs. And more relaxation is more energy flow and more inner strength and more healing! Yay!

I was very happy with my progress. However, it did not come by itself. I had to work for that. But first let's return again to Qi Massage.

I have once again had the pleasure to undergo Qi Massage. Twice! I love it when they are playing with your feet. Even more so when it's two people at the same time. Someone on the left, someone on the right and occasionally Ajahn comes in to give them some directions:
"Relax your shoulders, and then go from your center deeper into that point here"
"AW"
"Yes, that point is linked with the ankle and she is rather sensitive there."
"Grrrrr, are you kidding me?"
And then it was my turn. First a pile of mats had to be taken out so that I could stand on the right height and then the hands had to be folded around the 'victims' foot in a certain way. Like in the 7th static exercise, with the shoulders relaxed, relaxed in the elbows, pressure spread evenly over your fingers and don't press with your weight but with your

center. Aaaaaah! I'll have to practice a lot before I get that right!

And practicing I did:

Giving Qi Massage is easier said than done. Certainly when the massage tables are actually about 10 cm too high for me and I have to use a pile of mats to be able to get my hands in a comfortable position. Off course those mats have to be moved every time I move, from the legs to the back or from the left to the right. And at the same time I have to stay in my center. Right! But according to the one who had to undergo my 'experiments', it wasn't too bad. She said she could feel the tingling all the way to her ears. Amazing isn't it, you hold someone's feet in a certain way, make sure you're in your center, do nothing for the rest and she feels it in her ears.

The massage would be perfected further in the coming months and years. Not so much by giving a lot of massages but by going deeper into the knowledge of my own body. As a result, you know where find the different meridian points in another person faster and with more accuracy. However, some work had to be done on the knowledge of one's own body. Even today! I still learn new things about my body every day. I become more sensitive to what is going on. And because I no longer panic when there is pain or discomfort, I see it as a sign to go deeper. Therefore I can go to and deal with the root cause much quicker. And that is the beauty of this system. I am no longer dependent on doctors, pills, insoles, massages, osteopaths and whatever is out there. Yes but, I already hear you think, not everyone can spend 3 years in Thailand to learn that system. Fully agreed, but you don't have to. Just ask my mother. She only has her teacher-daughter with her for a few weeks a year (and then certainly we don't practice Qi Gong every day) but she sees huge improvements. How? She practices the first 4 of the 7 statics daily. That's the key. Being devoted. Just do it. It doesn't matter that it's not perfect. Because of the repetition her body knows what is coming, she doesn't need to think about it anymore and when I am there, it's easy for me to make very specific adjustments that she then can incorporate in her practice until that too becomes a habit. One that helps her. For example, the onset of arthritis in her fingers has been reversed, she no longer has neck pain and everyone thinks she is 10 years younger than she really is. In addition, she starts to understand that everything passes, including illness. Where she used to go to our GP for a common cold, she now takes ginger tea and lets her body do the healing work. And during her yearly examination he can only conclude that everything is okay. Better than last year even: "Your cholesterol level has dropped, for the third year in a row, good. And that blockage in your neck is also gone. " Thank you Medical Qi Gong!

But there is always something to learn and the process continues every day. I cannot say it better than with this Zen saying: You're perfect as you are, but there is always room for improvement. My ankle and my lower back begged for improvement.

And then suddenly the ankle made itself heard again. And it was f**king painful. I almost couldn't get out of bed and when I managed I was limping and felt 100 years old. Fortunately, I know by now that if I try to relieve the ankle by putting it under an angle instead of straight, it only makes things worse in the long run. It's not a solution. The only solution is to put the feet neatly in parallel, make the whole rolling motion and keep your weight in the middle when you walk (not wading like a duck). Do this very slowly and with your full attention for five steps and the pain decreases by leaps and bounds. To be honest it didn't vanish completely. So I expected that Ajahn would give me an acupuncture session but no. He thought this was a perfect opportunity to teach me how to use the pain and to further perfect the Qi Gong exercises. The pain indicates that I am not in my center in that particular position or movement. It indicates that I put the pressure too much on the inside or the outside of the ankle, or that I bring my weight too much forwards or backwards. Deep inside I cursed Ajahn a thousand times before I found the position/movement that didn't hurt but I now know 100 ways how I should not do it.

No acupuncture for the ankle, but for the back. And that while I have no problems there. I know, sometimes it's difficult to follow. Also for me. Too curious to just accept things, I asked the reasoning behind it. This is what I received as an answer.

"I read your body based on your movements, on top of that I felt during Qi Massage that you are empty in your back, there is no connection there. Your connection is only at the front. I know that acupuncture will accelerate the process of connecting that has begun with the Qi Gong exercises, I am weighing up whether it is worth accelerating that recovery."

Fair enough. Maybe it was also because I asked him if it could hurt to sleep on the floor. My bed is way too soft so I wake up in the morning with back pain (which disappears quite quickly). He said that sleeping on the floor is good so I rearranged my whole living space. The bed now serves as a very large sofa and I have made a floor bed from a number of blankets. Hurray, no more back pain in the morning!

I still sleep on a floor bed. Just a few blankets on the floor and your bed is made. Handy if you also use your studio to teach. Blankets in the closet and the room is ready to receive students. When those students hear that you are sleeping on the floor, their first question is usually: "Is it not hard? Don't you have any pain in your back in the morning? "No, my dear, this is the best present you can give your back. Outside of Qi Gong of course. And that's what we experienced. We? Yes Esra, a Turkish lady who is now teaching in Istanbul, joined us.

E sra already did 20 sessions a year and a half ago. She has decided to do Qi Gong intensively for three months to further work on her back problems. She has a similar back condition as I have but more severe, with complications to hips and legs. When she first started Qi Gong she was in tremendous pain and walking was very difficult. This has been addressed during the first 20 sessions and her subsequent practice at home but things can always be better. And that's why Luise has to teach us a new moving form called 'Fire Form'. The form should also improve my lordosis more. If the toes are an example, I am confident it will. The form, however, takes its toll on my back. I'm okay during practice of the form, it is only later, when we are practicing other things or when I am sitting at home on the sofa that I am in pain. Fortunately, I know that's a good thing. I know that it means that things are changing in those regions, because that's why we learn the form in the first place, to cure back problems. I just have to find a different, more aligned way of standing, sitting and walking because my 'old' way leads to pain. And I thought I knew my body because of my yoga practice... I guess not. Yes, I could (and still can) fold it in quite a few directions but making small subtle movements from my center? Forget it, my groins are too stiff for that. You wouldn't know it though when you see me putting my nose in between my knees.

Another sign that things are changing in the lower regions is the "happy re-entry" of my periods. I have been period free for 7 months. Until last month. A few small droplets. Oh no! I was so happy not to think about them anymore. The reason why they stayed away, you say? No idea and it really didn't matter to me. But okay, a few drops, you know, maybe it's only this time. Nope, this month it was a few big drops and just like last month it lasted only one day. Wondering what it will be next month. Ajahn had already warned me that they would come back when the energy in the back would begin to flow again. It's a natural elimination mechanism of the body. But then again, we could argue about that. It all depends on the theory you adhere to. Yoga says: no need to have your periods, better not, because with the blood you lose essential life energy. They even have certain poses that cause your periods to decrease or stay away completely. Maybe that was the reason they took a break in my case. Qi Gong says: periods are a natural elimination process of dead material. It's needed to purify your body. As long as it is not abundant, not (or little) painful and present, you don't change anything and you certainly don't do weird things to stop them. So, who do you believe? I am fortunate they don't have any effect on my daily life, but I don't want to stand in the shoes of the many women who are out for a couple of days every month.

More than 4 years later I can say the following about it. But first I have to share my personal history. I took the contraceptive pill from the age of 18 to the age of 27. Then I switched over to the Nuvaring® for 5 years and then switched again to the pill because of a slowly developing allergy to the ring. On my 34th I was sterilized with the help of laser, by choice and with great conviction. I have seen my periods evolve throughout the Qi Gong practice. First from a few drops for 1 day, over thick brown-black streaks for 3 days to how it is now: a minimal amount of bright red liquid, less than in my puberty, for about 3 days.

The day of ovulation and the day before the break-through of the periods I sometimes feel a nagging pain in the lower back. The PMS that started at least a week before the actual periods and that consisted of mood fluctuations and binge eating, has almost disappeared. Some months there can be a day just before my periods that I feel unusually depressed or on which I eat a whole bar of chocolate again. But nothing comparable with how it was 6, 7 years ago. So who do I believe now? I think it's a natural elimination process that you shouldn't try to stop. Prolonged, intense and painful periods can be balanced with Qi Gong. I have heard several students testify about their personal experiences with this. But what about the theory that together with the blood you lose your life energy? Theory that is supported by the fact that menstruation blood grows vegetables, fruit and flowers faster than ordinary water. Fertilizers, whatever animal they come from, do the same, don't they? Do you also want to stop that elimination process? When you have the chance, ask the people who suffer from constipation. I bet I know what they will tell you. No, no constipation here, but perhaps this is the ideal time to talk about the belly.

I want to talk about my belly. There are strange things going on. No, no diarrhea or other strange diseases. Then what? Well, my belly looks like I'm 6 months pregnant. You can already guess that I'm not really happy with that. Not to say that I find it terrible. But how come? Good question! I'll start from the beginning. For that I have to go back in time. About 30 years (Oh dear, I'm getting old!) At that time I was a rather fanatic gymnast. Training four times a week was very normal. And what did we get to hear every training session about a thousand times? "Suck in the guts" The result: sucking in my belly has become an automatism I no longer have to think about. It just happens without being aware of it. And it comes in handy, it gives you a nice body shape, right. Or maybe not? Because where does my arched back come from? In any case, I have built up a lot of muscles in the belly region. They were also strengthened by doing that strange belly thing during the yoga TTC. After three months of yoga, I had a fairly flat stomach. At least that was what I thought. Then you come to Qi Gong and the only thing you hear is: "Relax your belly, let it go". What? Are you kidding me?! I trained 36 years to pull in my stomach and now I have to do the opposite?! "Please explain to me why I suddenly have to let go of my belly. I hear nothing but pull it in and strengthen it because that is supposed to be good for your back and for your posture." A big grin, a finger pointing at my back and the announcement that they are clueless in the West. "Release it and you will understand it" and that was it. That was what I had to work with. Okay, it's a matter of trust I guess? So I consciously relax and let go of my stomach. I made a game of it. Every time I notice that I have sucked in my belly, I do the 'belly blob'. And that is about 17 times during a fifteen-minute meditation, 20 times during my ride to the clinic, 50 times during the class and 100 times during the rest of the day. And you know what? I start to understand it! Qi Gong is based on the fact that you don't need muscle to develop strength and speed. Just the opposite: Muscles are only blocking your inner strength (also called Qi or energy). What's more, as you get older, your muscles start to decay, a normal aging process. By doing muscle training, you are even going to speed up that process. It may seem on the outside that you are strong but actually they can easily push you over. I speak from experience: I can push my teacher over if he uses muscle power, but I can not move him a millimeter if he uses his Qi! The beauty is that I start to experience it myself now that I'm able to let go of my belly. By sucking it in I stopped the energy at the level of the solar plexus. And no matter how much I braced myself, a little push and I was out of balance, falling backwards. Now that I can let go of the belly, the energy goes to my center and I stay upright when I got pushed. Yiehaa!

Strength without using muscles! And what's more, the curve in my back slowly starts to look like a normal curve. Yiehaa! Power to heal my body! But that 6 months pregnant belly I'll have to put up with until the muscles I have built up there, understand that they are no longer needed and disappear to other shores and until I know how to find my center because I don't manage to do this every time yet. And that's the intention. That I can tap into that healing power at any time.

From the belly to the toes. When Ajahn told me during our very first conversation that my halux valgus on both feet would disappear, I didn't believe it for one bit. When after three weeks of practice he told me that my toes were changing, I didn't see any difference at all. "What the hell is he talking about? I don't see it, I see two big bumps and I see toes that are crooked." But what he saw, and I didn't, were not the big toes. He saw what was going on with the position of my little toes and then more specifically the second smallest from the right. That toe was crooked and always pressed against the middle toe so that I had to keep the nail very short as not to get blisters on that same middle toe. It was that second smallest toe he was talking about, it was that toe that had started to straighten. It started to dawn on me a lot later after I suddenly became aware that the nail didn't need any extra cutting and that I hadn't had blisters on the middle toe for a long time. After two months in my practice I started to see a difference myself. In the big toes. "Oh wow, look at this, this is really incredible, my big toe on the left is no longer on top of the next one! I have to take pictures of this!"

I took pictures my toes. I want to be able to prove black on white that I am not just imagining things, that there really is an energy that can heal your body. From now on every month I'm going to take a photo of my toes. Why my toes? The people who have ever seen them know. For the others: because they are crooked and because I want them to be straight. And if I can reverse this, everything is possible.

Everything is possible. The toes are straight! Admittedly, the left a bit more than the right. That right side stubbornly sticks to the last remnant of his old habits. Maybe it's because this way I can show my students from where I come. If everything is perfect, how are they going to believe me? I remember very well often telling Ajahn that it was easy for him to talk. "You have no weird curve in your back, you do not know what it's like." He did knew it because he had a severe back injury he healed with Qi Gong. Yet he is the first to admit that injuries often come and say hi especially if you are not paying attention. His back also did that, usually after a trip and handling heavy luggage. You saw him arriving in the clinic a little stiff. He left the teaching to one of his instructors and just joined the class. Half an hour later all stiffness was gone. That same grounding, being down to earth I too try to pass on in my classes. Qi Gong may solve your health problems, that does not mean that you are immune to them and that you will never again have any. After all, you are not a robot. It does mean that you have the tools to deal with it in your own hands. That you are no longer dependent on others or on chemical stuff. You have to learn to trust your own body and to let go of all concepts that you hold about it. When you don't do that you could encounter situations like the following.

A nd then Ajahn makes a student cry ... Not deliberately, if she had just done what he asked, nothing would have happened. But because she couldn't let go of her believe "my right foot is weak and I cannot use it to get up", she couldn't get up the first two times. And then the tears came. The moment she stopped fighting, let go of her limiting believe and just did what he asked, she got up perfectly. And she still did not want to see it for herself. She kept sticking to the idea that her foot was not strong enough, while she had just proven otherwise. Sometimes people are really strange creatures.

You can say that again. I am certainly no exception. Sometimes I look in the mirror and I still see that same curve in my back and am convinced that nothing has changed. Although I have all the proof that there is a huge difference with a few years ago. My backpack that now leans on my back instead of on my buttocks is the biggest proof. We are all human, we are all similar, yet we are all unique. And honestly admitted, I felt a bit special when I received a small gift from Ajahn with my birthday. It goes where I go. That's how I always have my Master with me.

For my birthday I got a gift from Ajahn. A traveling monk, 2cm high. It has two meanings. One of prosperity and one to remind me to stay on the right path, in the tradition of the Buddha. And then afterwards, oh irony, I have to hit him! When we practice martial art techniques among students, we don't touch each other. It's not the intention to hurt each other but to get the position of the hands, feet, knees, hips etc so that you are stable in case someone really would attack you and to create a reflex of defense instead of being shocked and freeze. The most important thing is to let the Qi flow so that your body can heal itself. Because we were three, we rotated so that each of us came to stand in front of Ajahn. And instead of doing what he told us to do, stepping backwards when you're attacked, he just stood still when it was my turn to attack him. My first reaction was to keep my hands to myself instead of continuing. He quasi indignant: "Don't stop!". Do you know how difficult that is? I needed at least 5 attacks before I dared to hit him and another 5 before I really dared to go for it. And even then it was very difficult. Would that be something feminine, shunning "violence"?

To ask questions about everything, would that also be something typically feminine? Or rather something typical for me? I asked a lot of questions. And not just about Qi Gong. Sometimes it was about some more practical things.

How do I put the daily 'routine' on paper so that it is a bit fun to read? Is it fun to know that every morning from the moment I'm getting out of my bed, after nature has done its work, I go sit on my butt, cross-legged, while a candle and an incense stick lighten up my room and that I close my eyes again? Not to sleep but to direct my full attention to my body posture. Ache in the back? Release the belly. Not yet gone? Tilt the pelvis. Thoughts already at breakfast? Come here naughty one, stay with your shoulders, neck, stomach, feet, etc. Is it fun to know that I already do that for 28 days? That there is a big difference in day to day concentration? That I sometimes give up after 10 minutes because my thoughts run rampant? That on other days it is suddenly 45 minutes later and I don't want to stop because I am so fascinated by the sensations in my body? That sometimes there is a silence and happiness coming over me that can not be described with words?

How can I explain that the exercises will not bore me? That I discover new sensations with every repetition? That one moment I find the right posture, the next moment I lose it again and only to find it again the next day or not at all. That, although it can not really be seen on the outside (except on the toes), my body is evolving. I feel that my groins are opening, that my shoulders are more relaxed, that I am more stable. But how do you explain that to people who are thousands of miles away from you?

I kept it up for hundred days in a row. One hundred days every morning sitting cross-legged and observing what happened in my body. I have suffered. I felt pain in places I had no idea that you could feel pain. I have cursed and cried. I have wondered a hundred times what I did to myself. But I have learned. I have learned what stagnation is. And how it leads to pain. I have learned what relaxation is. Not only physically but also mentally. I have learned how physical and mental relaxation go hand in hand and I have observed how pain disappears when you can relax and let go. Let go of your muscle tension, but also let go of your ideas about what "the right posture" is. What is center? What is straight? I have learned that sitting straight is something very different than the concept I had in mind about it. I still learn every day. I sometimes skip my meditation for a day or two, but due to a greater sensitivity to what is going on in my body, I discover more subtle layers. And although it sometimes seems that I come back to a point that I thought I had left behind me, I know that I stumbled upon the next, deeper layer. Unfortunately, pain is part of it. The sooner you can let go, the sooner your pain will disappear. How to let go, I cannot tell you. That, you have to find out for yourself. I can only tell you that if I can do it, you can do it too. Pain is something we are all afraid of, uncomfortable with, and of which we want to get rid of as quickly as possible. Yet pain has something to tell you. Do you want to hear it? Or do you want to suppress it with painkillers as soon as possible? Do you want another way to deal with pain? Are you ready for the discovery journey in your own body? You can do it step by step! Of course, all beginnings are difficult. There were also new challenges ahead of me. Learning a new form and starting to teach unpreparedly to name but two. Especially the teaching really came out of the blue.

And because my body learns from movement (not my words, Ajahn's words), I also got the second part of the 7 star form. Aaaahaaa, that's why I had to come half an hour earlier. During that half hour he could have warned me that he would put me in front of class. But no, he just says that we start sitting and that I have to prepare the mats after which he directs me to what is normally his place with the words: "You lead the meditation today." Huh, what, me? Euh. Okay then. Stress? Nah, no stress. Swallow. And that happened twice this week! I better be prepared because it will happen again. And it didn't stop with the meditation. A few days later, Ajahn was called away in the afternoon. He gave me phone call just before the lesson should start telling me that I had to tell Esra that she had to give Bellen a massage, that Shazia had to practice her form and that I should give Carmen the 7 statics. It felt a bit awkward to have to give instructions to Esra and Shazia, people who are my seniors in the practice. And that I, myself, still wet behind my ears, so to speak, had to teach a newcomer. It was an experience... One that taught me a lot. Especially how I should not do it.

The tone was set, my teaching career had started without my being aware of it. More of those unexpected teaching moments followed.

Before Ajahn leaves, he calls me to say that I have to teach chair exercises to our two male students. Okay, give me a minute to rub the sleep from eyes, take stools and direct those two to the kitchen. And then one of them takes my spot. Great, things started well. No, no I'm joking. It all went very smoothly. The only 'annoying' thing about teaching is that you concentrate less on your own body. You are more focused on your students. As a result, I suffered from lower back pain afterwards. An old habit that is returning and my body is now telling me: "Hey, that's not the way anymore!"

Thursday I was again a bit discombobulated when Ajahn, 15 minutes before the end of the open class in The Yoga Tree, directs me in front and says: "You give these three the first four movements of 7 star." These three are people who have been coming for years to Thursday class in The Yoga Tree. Uhm, okay then. After the first uneasiness had dissipated, I quite liked the experience. And coincidence or not, one of them had asked me before class if I wanted to be their teacher that day. Wish granted.

Yesterday the third teaching moment. And

now in French! You wouldn't believe how difficult it is to formulate the English wording that has been drilled in and comes without thinking in a different language. I know the words in French but they didn't come out. I even had to think three times before I could remember them in my mother tongue. Also today I had to stand in front of the class (small one, 3 students). Luckily this time it was in English, matter of giving my brain a little rest on a Sunday.

That same brain conjured up quite some images when Ajahn gave my a broom.

I thought I had seen just about everything. That was without taking my teacher into account. He put a broom in my hands after class! When I told him a while ago that I had enjoyed the bamboo training and would like to do it again, I definitely had something else in mind.

Let me explain: In August there were a number of afternoons that I was the only student. During those afternoons I had three classes with a long bamboo stick of about two meters. I had to stand opposite of Ajahn, our sticks crossed in the air. He made circles with his stick and my stick had to follow his without being separated from each other.

It sounds simple, it's terribly difficult! After that, the sticks were crossed on the ground and we alternately knocked the other his stick away. Of course not just like that, there is a technique you have to use: swing from your center and with your Qi instead of with your muscles. If you don't do that your arms, your back, your legs, your entire body basically starts to hurt. The goal was to make me understand that I was not able to put power behind my swings because of using too much muscle. That much more power can be gained from relaxing your muscles and moving from your center. Although I suffered a great deal of pain, I thought it was super fun to do. I already saw myself, as in the Chinese fighting films, alla "Crouching Tiger, Hidden Dragon" or "House of the Flying Daggers" going around swinging with a bamboo stick and knocking the air out of all the bad guys. Yes, I know, a lot of imagination. When he called me after class, he said that he had thought of my bamboo training. He pulled out a broom (one that witches fly on), estimated the height and said it was perfect for my size. I must have given him a strange look because he laughed. "If I teach you bamboo, it'd better be useful" was his comment. He has shown me how to hold the broom and how to sweep (it is indeed the same as with the stick) and from tomorrow on I have to sweep the courtyard. 5 or 10 minutes would do. I really felt like Karate Kid at that moment. He got paint brushes, I got a broom. Until there my imagination, no swinging sticks, I will have to face the bad guys with a broom. Will I make it into the movies?

So after a demonstration and the encouraging words : "Figure it out, you can do it." I busied myself with my whisk broom in between classes on Monday, Tuesday and Friday. I have yet to find the trick. No two minutes in and I already had pain in my lower back. So I changed hands, to no avail. Yet another change, trying different position of the hands, different position of the feet, back, knees, hips. Oh man, it still hurts, I give up. That courtyard will never get clean. Especially not when a storm comes over Chiang Mai at night. You no longer saw that I had done anything. Oh well, getting the courtyard clean is probably not the goal anyway, the goal is to learn to move from my center. Whether that is during Qi Gong exercise or with a broomstick in my hands (beware, witch Ils is coming, make sure you're out of my way) does not matter. Unfortunately I haven't found that magical center yet. That's what my lower back tells me for sure!

In the meantime I am the proud owner of a real witches broom, of Greek manufacture this time, and

I finally got the trick. No more back pain while I sweep my studio. Nothing has come of the bamboo training with "real" sticks. The clinic became increasingly popular, so other priorities were pushed to the forefront. Some things had to be arranged for myself too. After a year of life-changing discoveries I really couldn't go back to a job I did because "I had to do something" and because it provided me with a good standard of living. I just couldn't give up Qi Gong like that. I wanted to develop the changes I felt and saw in my body and yes, those few tastings of teaching also asked for more. So there had to be flown back to Belgium to quit a job and rent out a house. In addition to a hundred other things that made that three week in for my liking ice-cold Belgium were over before I knew it.

PART III

The Wonder of Qi Gong

About teaching and letting go

(Feb 2015- Sep 2017)

7. TEACHING, LETTING GO AND HEALING

Was I starting level 2 or 3 of the Instructor Training at the beginning of 2015 after the Belgian intermezzo? I lost count. It was of little importance. After 7 months of continuous practice, I began to see what I have already mentioned. That this system of Medical Qi Gong lends itself rather difficult to be divided into levels, that it's a lifelong learning process and that the experiences, although similar, are very individual. I still didn't have a career in Qi Gong in mind when I arrived back in Chiang Mai after my Belgian in between. While in Belgium my dad recovered from the placement of a knee prosthesis with adapted Qi Gong exercises, the same ones that the crippled man had done, I just wanted to devour everything there was to learn about Qi Gong. The learning process, however, was playing out very differently than I was used to. I am someone who acquires knowledge fairly easily. I only need to read or hear something a few times and it's in my head. Especially if it's a subject that interests me. Qi Gong is a topic that interests me but Qi Gong doesn't work with knowledge. Qi Gong works with repetition, a lot of repetition. Qi Gong works with letting go of knowledge. And with surrender. You can hardly express letting go and surrender in words and that is why it's often referred to as "not". The favorite expression of my teacher: "Don't go there." It made me utterly frustrated. But now that I teach myself, I understand that there are things you simply cannot explain, for which you should only use vague words so that students don't pin down on the words. We absolutely want to avoid that. We want to leave our brain out of the equation as much as possible, we want to understand the language of our body. And that's a completely different language, one that refused to follow my normal learning process. Leaving my brain aside turned out to be a big challenge. A further deepening in Qi Massage helped me with that. Although students come to the Qi Massage course to learn massage, they soon discover that massage is only secondary. The priority is finding your own center. When you are there, you can give a good massage. Not by using muscle strength. As a recipient, you feel that difference. I myself have become very picky when it comes to massages. But I'm getting ahead of myself.

It was time for my first official Qi Massage course. Two super-interesting weeks. The strange thing is that you don't have to do anything other than being relaxed, being in your center and keeping your hands in the right places. Then the energy automatically flows between the giver and the receiver. And the recipient can (but need not) feel that as a kind of electricity that passes through his body. Being relaxed and being in your center is of course the art. A difficult art. Only when holding another body you will become aware of all the places in your body where you still hold tension! Relaxed in my shoulders? Yeah in my dreams! All in all, it was not too bad with the tensions. I even managed to bring one of our students in balance. When we started she had a headache, it was as if her shoulders were on fire, so much heat shone from them, and her feet were ice-lumps. After about a half-hour massage her feet were warm, the heat in her shoulders had dropped to a normal body temperature and she said her headache had diminished. Wow, I was really impressed. It was tangible! Not something imagined. Of course I couldn't have done this without my 7 month practice as a basis. This is not something you can learn in a short course. Thankful that I can further explore it now!

There was also further exploring of teaching. Not because I wanted to, but because according to Ajahn it was the right time. Because it's another way to turn off your brain. Because it complements your own practice. Your students are your best teachers. They hold a mirror for you. They give you the chance to check whether the 'deviation' you see in them is also present in yourself. What can be quite pronounced with them can be very subtle in your own body. In this way I still learn to recognize more subtle layers of stagnation in my own body. So here is a big bow and a sincere thank you to all students who have enriched my path and are still enriching it. And although the beginning was difficult, witness the next two posts, I would not want to change it for anything in the world.

Qi Gong was mainly about teaching. Ajahn put me in front of class a number of times and gave me feedback afterwards and answered my questions. He also asked me to give some of the classes while he is in Indonesia for a few days. I like it but it is also very difficult because those who are now practicing in the clinic are no longer beginners. Sometimes I see things that I think are not quite right, but I have no idea how to adjust that. Ajahn will be bombarded with questions when he comes back.

What a week! I have been teaching 5 times! Let's say that it's something completely different than being a student yourself. Fortunately, we were only four or five. That was enough to start. I couldn't manage more than cycling home, grab a bite and flop down in the hammock. But I've learned a lot. And noticed that I finally start to understand a number of things that Ajahn tried to explain me in the beginning. I recall him saying about a 100 times while l did a certain movement: "You go to the side, go to the front, you go to the hips, go to the feet. You will create stagnation in the hips." By the way, stagnation is no good for nothing, it only gives rise to all kinds of conditions, in the extreme even to osteoporosis. I didn't understand what is he was talking about, I was certain that I was going to the front! Now I see it, now I understand. It is a subtle difference but clear when the body gets it. Now I can feel the difference between going to the side or going to the front, but the person I was trying to explain it to didn't understand it, just like I didn't in the beginning. To see that, made me feel her, I understood her frustration because I had gone through it myself. But more than that, I understood that I still have a long way to go because it's so easy to relapse into old habits. Just a moment of being with my thoughts somewhere else and there I went to the side again.

In addition to more body awareness, changes were also taking place in other areas. The first person who made me aware of this was Carmen.

A week and a half ago, Carmen suddenly appears in the clinic. What a nice surprise! Carmen attended two weeks of classes in November 2014 and now she was suddenly back! After half a day she told me she thought I had changed so much in the four months she hadn't seen me. Not only physically but also mentally. She told me that I was much more open, less rigid in my thinking and more tolerant towards other people. Wow! I was speechless. Qi Gong apparently goes deeper than just the physical!

Indeed, slowly but surely changes occurred and that intangible and sometimes incomprehensible letting go became less elusive. Perhaps physical tension is partly a consequence of mental tension? Of unconscious patterns that must first be seen and recognized? Or maybe it's the other way around? You can at least say that the physical and the mental are connected. But because the mental is so volatile, it is much easier to work with the physical. Our bodies show stubborn patterns much more easily than our minds do. Your posture, your way of moving are fairly consistent over time. Your thoughts, on the other hand, can change from one second to the next, making it very difficult to recognize ingrained habits and reactions. It's already difficult for us to recognize ingrained habits in our body if we are not told, let alone in the mind. That's why in Medical Qi Gong we work with our body. The more we become aware of unhelpful patterns in our bodies, the more we can also recognize mental patterns. I got a taste of it in 7 star part 2.

The movements of the second part of the 7 star form I was taught a while ago but there has never been time to go deeper into it. Until now. Due to circumstances, the last half of the afternoon class turned out to be a private class for me. Well! I've definitely been brought back to earth. I thought I was doing a good job, but old habits are apparently very stubborn and very much alive in "new" movements. And it is not only the physical habits that come up again, but also the mental habits (frustration that I cannot get it right the first time, wanting to have it all under control) are clearly arising. The biggest difference with a few months ago is that now I am aware that this is happening. I can laugh at it instead of letting it drag me along. Like "Okay, here I go again!" And from the moment I see it, the frustration disappears. Where it used to linger hours after the class because I just did not realize what I was doing (condemning myself because I didn't get it right the first time), it now disappears in the light of my awareness. So yes, Carmen was right, it were not only physical changes.

These changes continued and were, in my opinion, accelerated during my first Qi Gong Retreat (April 2015) in Bali. I didn't know what to expect, only that it would be an intense experience. Ten days from morning to evening doing Qi Gong. In the meantime I have done 7 retreats in Bali and I still don't know what to expect because each retreat has its own focus which emerges organically depending on the students who are present. The practice space, a Thai Buddhist temple, is the same, as well as the place where we sleep, every time Ajahn's wife conjures up the most delicious meals on our plates, but the duration and the content of each retreat is different. That you encounter yourself and your stubborn physical and mental habits goes without saying. I remember vividly that during my first retreat I had it on day 7. I was done, it was enough, I could take no more. Then letting go comes in. How do you do that? I am sure that some tears have flowed, that I bit Ajahn's head off a couple of times, and that pages of my journal has been scribbled full. Yet it was fascinating to notice progress both in myself and in my fellow students. While the first retreat was mainly about my own practice, the following retreats were more about how to teach. I also noticed that in every subsequent retreat the I-have-had-it feeling occurred much later or not at all. I could more and more align with what happened there. Open, let go, flow. After the second retreat (sept 2015) I shared the following on the blog. And it perfectly reflects what was going on in my world.

It was fun, instructive, difficult, tiring, at times stressful, but above all mind-expanding and worth every effort. I learned so much, evolving in my own practice and in my teaching. Learning to sit still for more than 2 hours, learning to keep my mouth shut when I don't immediately understand something (very difficult for me), teaching in a different way, learning to feel the energy of the group, seeing myself and my automatic reactions and trying to nip them in the bud (still a long way to go), trying to understand Ajahn when he (according to me) speaks in riddles again. For the sake of clarity, he doesn't speak in riddles, it's I who cannot or does not want to understand/accept what he is saying. After letting it sink in overnight it usually becomes clear. Sometimes it takes much longer. It all depends on how stubborn I want to stick to my own ideas. A number of other things also suddenly clicked. "Ah, that's what you mean by 'connect the backline'." I hope that these flashes of insight will stay with me because I have already noticed that I lose those clicks and go back to my old ways. I need the same click several times before it sticks.

The series of sensations was there before that second retreat and just continued after it. I couldn't do anything other than observe and undergo. Whether that was pleasant or not. Unfortunately, I didn't have a say in that. The first step to change and healing is always becoming aware and not fighting it. Just breathe through it. You can do more than you think. Those sensations, by the way, still continue every day. They are less extreme, more subtle than in those early days. They will continue until the day I die. Do you find that discouraging? Quite the opposite! Your body is different every day, every moment. Qi Gong teaches you to deal with this changing reality. To let go of what was yesterday and to look for a new balance. Your body just wants to help you with that, so that you don't end up in patterns that don't benefit your health. And sometimes it doesn't feel pleasant at all.

Early morning was a period of welcoming. Saying hi to fatigue, to a back that hurted, to ankles that where cramping up, questioning almost everything and wanting to crawl back under the covers (if they had been necessary). What the hell was that? In the afternoon, things got better mentally. Physically lots of things were still happening. Strange, never-felt sensations came and went, pains came and went. My body seemed to go through its four seasons in one day. The hammock gently caught it and didn't need long to lull it to sleep.

From one extreme to the other. And that in a few days.

It was the most memorable day so far in my Qi Gong practice. Never before did I experience all these things that were going on in my body. Was that the sense of energy flow? If yes, give me more please! At one point it felt as if I were growing, as if I were being stretched out. It felt as if there was more space in my whole body. Everything felt much less heavy, the curve in my back became smaller and it felt like a load was being lifted from my shoulders. Afterwards my 7 star form became much smoother, things I've been fighting with for weeks (your foot stays behind, you hold it in your knees, from your center instead of from your hips, ...) all of the sudden disappeared like it was nothing. I loved it!

If one part went more or less well, then another part needed some work. The thighs were not the only cause of my arched back, also the buttocks had something to do with it.

My posture has changed a lot, but in certain positions I still automatically and unconsciously lift my buttocks. Those years of gymnastics have left their mark. And those marks I now have to erase because by tensing my buttocks, my back arches. And let that be the very thing I have been trying to change during the last 10 months! At one point I managed to really be in my center and to relax those buttocks. Wow, what a nice feeling! As if I had no buttocks anymore! Much lighter but much more grounded. And a feeling of more space in my back. Unfortunately, I couldn't replicate it again. And the more I tried, the less it worked of course. Talking about learning patience, click number 2 and 3 will come. I think I start to get what the Buddhists mean when they say that you are not the owner of your body. It just does what it wants, when it wants. Helping it off in the right direction is the only thing you can do.

After the first retreat, Ajahn focused more and more on learning to teach. Our most senior instructor would do a tour for a month or six and trusted me with her weekly classes at The Yoga Tree, a center for dance, yoga and wellness in the heart of Chiang Mai. D-day: May 19, 2015. A month to get ready and be prepared. So many times I was unexpectedly put in front of the class. And there were a lot of revelations for me.

At times Ajahn was explaining things when he suddenly said: "Ils, now you guide." It is difficult to make that transition from student to someone in front of the class. I received feedback afterwards. How I could improve things. Or he asked me to pay more attention to how he builds a class. "Ooh, there is structure in that? That's been thought about? Really?" It seems as if he is pulling it all out of the hat on the spot. And partly that's also the case. What he does depends on the people who are there and what they need. But how he does it, how he conveys it, there is a logic in that. That was new to me.

By now I have seen several times how Ajahn prepares someone to teach. It improves my teaching because I did not get the subtler clues from the first time. In addition, I have also seen that we all go through the same thing. Explaining too much, going into details too much, expecting too much from your students. I sometimes catch myself doing it still. Also never send a message with compliments from one of your students to your teacher.

I f I have to believe him, I am a "natural teacher". He even sent me a message via Facebook to say that he had really enjoyed the class and that he was impressed by my clear, structured explanation and structure of my lesson. Honestly, I never prepare my classes. But it's nice to hear from someone who has been in front of a class full of school children for years. I forwarded the message to Ajahn. Not a good idea. The next day he put my head back on straight: "Don't do it like that, stand there, pay attention, speak louder, not too loud, ..." Okay, okay, I understood. No chance of letting it go to my head. After that it seemed that Ajahn wanted to see how stable, literally, I am in my Qi Gong exercises. Getting a good push between my shoulders on the unexpected, him trying to pull my hands apart, testing my defense while three men were watching (their faces afterwards, divine!) A few times an approving nod, once even a sincere "gooood". Then you think you're doing a good job only to get 700 new adjustments to your form two minutes later. Sigh. But it does mean that it was good because otherwise I wouldn't get those new adjustments, then he would just keeps hammering on the old ones. Discouraging? Frustrating? No, not at all! Only if you forget that it is good to get adjustments.

As if being tested by Ajahn was not enough, Life gave me the ultimate chance to prove to myself the power of Qi Gong once and for all. It served me a broken elbow. A motorcycle came from behind a car with great speed and hit the front wheel of my bicycle. I caught the impact of the fall with my left hand. At first I thought it wasn't too bad. A few scratches.

But probably the adrenaline suppressed the pain because as the evening progressed, it got worse and I couldn't straighten out my left arm anymore. Shit, that was also what happened about 25 years ago but on the right side. I was convinced that it was fractured. I wanted to wait until the next day because there was no swelling, maybe it was nothing. The night was long and interrupted. The next day still no swelling but with every small movement a sharp pain and the range of motion was even less than the evening before. I used a scarf to make a sling and took a songthaaw to the hospital. An hour later I got the verdict: a fracture in the head of the radius (one of the two bones in the forearm). They wanted to put me in a cast, but I remembered far too well what a hell those six weeks cast were and even more what a hell the physiotherapy was afterwards. I was like: "wowowowow, wait a minute!" A number of WhatsApp messages were exchanged with Ajahn who was in Jakarta at the time asking what was the best for me to do. Of course he didn't want to give an unambiguous answer:

"I don't have your arm, ask questions: how bad is the fracture, what can you do with it, why do they want a cast, use your logic, don't panic, be present."

Don't panic, easier said than done. "Okay, Ils, slow breaths, in and out. And use your brain, you have it for a reason."

I left the hospital without a cast. A tight elbow band and a scarf as a sling were all medical devices that I used during my recovery. No painkillers. Not that first night, nor after that.

My body let me know very clearly which movements I could and could not do. As long as I kept everything still, there was no problem. So now let's test what Qi Gong really can do.

Oh I have tested it. I've squeezed out everything that could be squeezed out. I tested the power of Qi Gong until there was nothing more to test. I started 36 hours after the accident. What a journey it was.

The testing has begun. With meditation. In the Medical Qi Gong meditation posture, we intend among other to bring the energy to the fists. Let me see if I can do that. Challenge number 1: how do I bring the wrist in the right position when it is painful to turn the arm?
"Aw, not like that."
"Hmm, I cannot use yang line. Okay, let's do it from yin line then."

"Hmm, that works. Wooow! Cool!"

Challenge number 2: making fists.

"Aw! shoot! I again used yang line. Yin line Ils! Okay, that's better."

30 minutes later I was seriously impressed: my fingers, which were as bit swollen and stiff, were back to normal and the freedom of movement was slightly larger. Beautiful!

In the afternoon I tried to do 7 static nr 1 to 3. Just once to experience.

"Hmm, still a bit too painful."

The next day the test continued again with meditation. No more pain, I knew now how to do the movements. The arm also straightened out more as the meditation progressed.

Test day No 3: No more problems during the meditation. Everything is back as it was before the fracture (incredible!) So time to go a bit further: 7 static No. 1 to 6. Where on the first day of testing certain movements were still very painful, not so much anymore on the third test day. Where on test day 1 I could barely get my arm past a 90 degree angle, on day 3 it could already go past 135 degrees! Wonderful! However I decided to skip 7 static No. 7 because leaning on the fingertips is just a little too early. And what about my 7 star form? As long as I work from yin line it goes well, when I use yang line (and that's happening a lot because years of gymnastics taught me to move mainly from my yang line) there is pain. Interesting what a broken elbow can teach you: a new way of moving where there is more balance between yin and yang, a faster way of healing (imagine that I had been in a cast with no possibility to move!) and even more trust in the Qi Gong system.

On test day 4 (day 5 after the accident) I was able to do the first 6 exercises without feeling any pain. Wow! Would I dare to do No 7, the leaning on the fingertips? Let's try once. "Hmmm, it's still a bit too early." But it strengthened me in the belief that I could teach my Yoga Tree class. And yes, I did it. I was teaching class one week after the accident. A small class, with three people and I improvised a bit because I couldn't do all the warm-up exercises yet. After that class I took a songthaaw to the clinic. Ajahn was back and wanted to hear my story. When he saw the scrapes on my hand, his comment with a big smile on his face was: "Good fall, you missed the center of your hand only by one centimeter. Better next time, practice some more 7 static number 2 and 3." I think my eyes were shooting fire! Which off course made him laugh even more. To give him credit, he was genuinely worried and wanted to see what I could and couldn't do with my arm. We did 7 statics and he seemed surprised at my recovery.

"Pain?"

"No."

"That pain?"

"No."

"And that?"

"No."

"Oh"

Hihi, my turn to laugh. Truth is, I've had 5 days to figure out how to use that yin line.

And with that the normal routine had been restored. I did not, however, started cycling again. That had to wait a bit longer.

Day 10 was a real test day! Attacking and defending with a broken arm. Fortunately, the person in front of me had compassion with me and didn't use his full power. But because of this practice I experienced that as long as I was relaxed and connected, things were okay. I didn't even feel pain. It only took a bit of time to find that relaxed and connected mode. I figured that if I could attack and defend myself, I also could go by bike. Another test (day 11: the bike test). Yes, it was okay but I had to be very careful. The bumps were still a bit painful. But cycling with one hand is feasible too, right.

And then it was time for the real test: day 14 a new X-ray. How that turned out? According to the doctor, the fracture was already healed for 60%. He told me that he would like to see me again within three weeks and that I still had to keep the arm in a sling (yes yes) that I should not move too much (no no) and that I had to take it easy (yes yes). I didn't dare tell him that I didn't use the sling anymore since five days, that I had come to the appointment with the bicycle and that I had been doing Qi Gong exercises from day 2 on. I couldn't turn his whole world upside down, could I? He already looked at me as if I was crazy when I asked him if I could return the pills he had given me. Heavy painkillers and an anti-inflammatory that I really didn't need! There was no swelling, so no inflammation. Why then for God's sake would I need anti-inflammatory drugs? And the pain told me which movements I could and couldn't do. Instead of suppressing it with painkillers, I listened to it and used it to get to understand my body better. Actually, it is unbelievable that they want to put you in a cast for 6 weeks, which means that you have to go through physiotherapy for at least another 6 weeks to regain your normal range of motion. In less than three weeks I did 90% of my normal movements completely pain free. I am convinced. There is no possibility they ever get me into a cast again. Hopefully I'm spared from such a situation arising again. And hopefully my experience makes you think twice before you agree with a cast. Your body can do more than you think!

You can be sure of that! And also be sure that you are your best doctor. As Hippocrates said: "If you are not your own doctor, you are a fool." That was definitely apparent from the discrepancy between what the doctor told me 5 weeks after the accident and my reality.

Yesterday I went back for the last X-ray and this is what the doctor said: "It's healing. you don't need to come back anymore, but you can not lift, push and pull during the next month."
"Uhuh."
I have been lifting the 20 liter water bottles for two weeks. I pull open the heavy iron gate of the clinic and close it without any problems or pain. What is occasionally a bit painful is putting some weight on it. We have a stretching exercise in which we sit on the floor and lean on the hands. If I don't do it consciously, I still feel a little pain. But everything else is okay. Bending, straightening, turning as if nothing ever happened! And that after 5 weeks! Amazing, isn't it?

As if the healing of a broken elbow was not enough to confirm and strengthen my faith in the power of Qi Gong, I was presented with an injury far worse on the day of my last hospital visit. Not for myself, but Kathy could be an older version of myself. When I met her she was a Buddhist nun. In the meantime she has handed back her robes and lives and works in Japan now. We have had many adventures together, inside and outside of Qi Gong. However, I will never forget our first meeting.

Yesterday I got a visit from a nun in the clinic. One that was as short as I am but she had a dislocated vertebra. "Normal" medicine could do nothing more for her than to stuff her with drugs that didn't help. Even morphine and cortisone did nothing to relieve her pain that radiated towards her leg because the sciatic nerve was pinched. An operation was too expensive and even if she could afford it, she wasn't keen on it either. To give her some relief she uses a corset to support her back and keep it from moving. Because Ajahn is in Indonesia, I am dependent on my own judgment. Which is a bit frightening with such a serious injury. When I asked her to take off her corset so that I could look and feel, it was with somewhat trembling legs. But so interesting. I could easily feel the place of the dislocation. It was a dent in her spine, the muscles around it were very tight and the skin was hot. Okay, let's see what we can do. Just standing upright was already very difficult for her, even after the adjustments to her posture. Also, sitting on a chair turned out to be very painful but that improved after she understood the principle of sitting correctly (on the feet instead of on the back and the buttocks). Because she even slept with the corset on, I showed her how she could lie on her side to open her back and relieve the pain. She was surprised that she could do it without pain. I then gave her a Qi Massage of about twenty minutes. Remarkable that afterwards the dent had become smaller, the muscles were relaxed and the heat was completely gone! She herself was pleasantly surprised and will return tomorrow. I am so grateful that I'm allowed and able to do this: helping people find their own healing mechanisms. And the deeper I go into my own practice, the better I can do that. So if on a lesser day, when nothing seems to work and I wonder why I do this again, I will think of that little nun. And remember it.

The recovery process of Kathy was not always straightforward. What is not exceptional with Qi Gong, but when she shuffled in, nose almost touching the floor for her fourth session, I didn't know what to think at all.

My heart skipped a couple of beats. This cannot be because of Qi Gong exercises and Qi massage, can it?

No, she had had an acupuncture session the day before with someone who apparently didn't understand the yin/yang philosophy. The person had just stabbed needles on her painful side. And there you go, all the balance that I had tried to obtain with the Qi Gong and the Qi massage all of a sudden gone. Because in her condition she was not able to do any exercises, I just put her on the massage table and after an hour and a half she stood straight up again. She has wisely decided to cancel her next acupuncture session and to rely on the system we use. And when he returned from Indonesia, Ajahn saw that it was good. He felt that she didn't need acupuncture, the knowledge of the exercises I had given her and some time should be enough to make her like new.

She is completely recovered, her back shows no trace of what happened, all vertebrae are neatly back in place. Later on, I helped her to recover from a fall on her tailbone and a knee injury. All these experiences made her decide to spend 6 months in the clinic to go deeper into the TQH Medical Qi Gong system. Somewhat later, when I already had left Chiang Mai behind me, she took private lessons for two weeks as a reminder.

When I look back now, I realize that 2015 was a very intense year. One in which I learned a lot. Not only on the level of Qi Gong but also on a personal level. Both physically and emotionally there were so many changes. A back that slowly but surely lost its unnatural curvature, toes that were straightening out more and more. Daring to write down on the blog that I sometimes too felt lost, that I was openly angry with Ajahn. Yet at that moment, it was all pretty normal and I didn't give it a second thought. To me, life went its normal course.

I try to flow with it. That is: going to sleep when I am tired, whether at 9 pm or at midnight (or falling asleep at 8 pm in the hammock, waking up at 11 pm and then moving to my bed) and getting up when I wake up. On most days that would be between 5.30 and 6.00 am. Sometimes even at 4.30 am. The first thing I still do after getting up is sitting on my yoga mat in a cross-legged pose and meditating for half an hour to three quarters of an hour. The conversations that take place in my head are hilarious at times. Or the same song always comes up, or I start playing back the past, or my shopping list comes up. I am there and watch it. And wonder how many selves I have... and who/what is the real me? And sometimes there is silence, the conversations in my head gone. Wonderful!

Is it only for that silence that I meditate? No, I don't. Through meditation I can better understand in daily life that thoughts are just thoughts, feelings just feelings, that they arise and dissolve without me having to react. I am less entrained by the inevitable waves of thoughts and emotions that arise and often have nothing to do with the reality of the moment. And when I get sucked in in the story, I can get out more easily by just seeing what is real, instead of what goes on in my head.

The rest of the day is filled with Qi Gong. If it's not being a student then it's teaching. And I love to do both. Teaching gives such satisfaction because you see people change. Their posture becomes more relaxed and their pains disappear. With a more relaxed posture, they often get a more relaxed view of life too. So beautiful to be able to experience that evolution up close. And being a student is both nice and challenging. Nice because I can concentrate on my own body and not have to think about others. At the same time it's challenging because deeper layers are being unearthed each time. Or how my body needs thousands of repetitions to release a certain tension that causes pain. The first 1000 repetitions are to feel that there is tension, the second 1000 is to really feel the pain and the third 1000 is to get the it right, the motions as well as the relaxation. If all goes well, the next 1000 are needed to fully understand and pass it on. And then it starts all over again with the next movement because habits are difficult to unlearn. Give me a little bit a different motion and there is that old bad habit again. The cycle starts over. Luckily I find it unbelievably fascinating.

Now, I have to admit that there are really times when I desperately think: "I will never be able to do this, how can I teach if I cannot do it myself." Sometimes I get so frustrated that I let Ajahn have it.

"My back hurts and you just say relax, but how can I relax, there must be something I can do! Should I be more forward, should I go more to the back, WHAT?! Don't go there, let go, what does that mean? How do you do that? HOW?!"

These times although it looks like I'm fighting with everything and everyone, I really only fight with myself. With my body and my mind. I want it to be different than it is. And the moment the fighting stops, tada, the light goes on! I know that the less I fight, the faster I get it. And yet, and yet. It seems that I have to come to a certain boiling point before I can let it go, before I can surrender. And there you go, no back pain during the exercises today, I had given up, I surrendered.

Incredible and so applicable in everything I
do. Go with the flow for the least problems. If
I want it my way, olala.

You can see this as a clear example of how fighting with what is leads to suffering. Emotional and
physical suffering. Not only for yourself but also
for others. My body gave me the chance to become
rooted in the here and now. To bring my awareness to
something that is real. Instead of ceasing that chance
I resisted it. I saw it as something to get rid off as
fast as possible. I wanted to solve it with my mind.
But mind is actually part of the problem. It takes you
away from the here and now, it takes you into an illusion, a story that it has crafted. That story told me
that Ajahn had to tell me exactly what I had to do
to get rid off that "damn" back pain. It told me that
his guidance was way too vague, that it was of no
use at all. It made me accuse him of not having one
empathic bone in his body. My little show of temper,
which probably hurted me more than him because
he understood where it came from, contrary to myself, took me even further away from what was really
going on. Namely, me believing a story my mind conjured up. I wrote back then that it seemed that I had
to get to a certain boiling point before I could let go.
Luckily things also changed there. I realise faster that
my mind is making up stories again. And I can step
out of them more easily by going to my body. By con-
centrating on my breath for instance. Focussing on
what's happening in my body prevents me reaching

that critical boiling point thus breaking the cycle of unconscious reactions. To be honest, I'm just human and far from perfect. Some stories are very alluring and I still can be entranced by them. But practice makes perfect.

8. CHOOSING MYSELF

While I was wondering how I to be able to teach when feeling inadequate to perform the exercises myself, reality gave me the answer. Ils, you can teach perfectly well because look, you are doing it! You run the clinic when Ajahn is in Indonesia, you attract new students who are not running off screaming and you are guiding and helping a nun with a dislocated vertebra. What more do you want? Well, between you and me, perfection. I wanted perfection, I wanted everything to go smoothly, painless and perfect from the first time. Unfortunately, it doesn't work that way. Qi Gong is a process. One that never stops and where perfection doesn't exist. I still struggle with some of the exercises, even during my classes. Which shows my students that I'm not superwoman, that even after more than 4 years I too have to search for my center. Time and time again. This is not something that you get in 10 or 20 sessions. Please be patient with yourself!

While 2014 was the year in which everything started and 2015 the one in which I grew exponentially in understanding, I like to call 2016 the year of deepening. My practice and teaching became more stable. There were fewer doubts whether what I did was good enough. I also felt much less the need to put everything down in writing. The blog posts came out more irregularly and when they appeared they were less centered around the whole Qi Gong experience. Only the things that appealed to me or amazed me where deemed worthwhile to share. In addition, I began to understand that words are not always the best way to convey something. They can create expectations that stop your personal evolution. I heard fellow students talk about energy flow and sensations that they felt. All they got from me was a blank stare. I really didn't understand what they were talking about. Yes, I sometimes felt something as you could read in the previous chapters. Usually those sensations were short-lived and I could not reproduce them. Ajahn always reassured me that I shouldn't worry about it and not focus on it either. He even said that it could be a disadvantage because instead of focusing on your posture and your center, you start to focus on regaining a certain sensation. A sensation that is not always a sign of being in your center. I remember very well the next incident while we were practicing 7 star part 2. Suddenly one of the students is told: "Yes, that's it, you're perfectly in center right now!" Her reaction was an astonished: "But I don't feel anything at all." Indeed, you don't have to feel anything at all. It is possible, it is allowed and it's there sometimes, and sometimes it isn't. Just observe it. You can not compare two days with each other, they are always different. You can not compare two repetitions, your body is different, it has learned, so don't go looking for something that was there yesterday or a moment before. Stay with what is showing up now. And that applies not only to Qi Gong but also to life in general. After 3 busy weeks in Belgium where we welcomed my brothers firstborn into the family, I was looking for some rest. Life gave me the opposite.

What a hectic week! And it seems that it will continue for a while. Medical Qi Gong Level 1 has started. Suddenly 6 extra people in the clinic. Meanwhile, the "regular" classes for instructors and patients took place on the terrace or in the kitchen or in both if we were too many to fit into the room... I had to be flexible. Ajahn asked me to follow the Level 1 at certain times, at other times he calls me away from that class to the kitchen to show me how he adapts the exercises for an ALS patient. At again other times I had to go to the terrace to practice 7 star with the other instructors. Then in the afternoon he asked me to assist with acupuncture which means taking the needles out of the package and carefully watching where Ajahn puts them. In addition, there are the Tuesday and Thursday classes that I teach in The Yoga Tree and which were busy this week (9 and 12 people).

On Friday morning I got confirmation from two Yoga Tree students that they want to start Monday with 20 sessions, I hear Friday afternoon from Ajahn that he has to go to Indonesia for another five days. A day later he had already left.

Life not only kept me busy but also gave me astonishment and confirmation of the power of Qi Gong.

I would like to share something wonderful. I have long been convinced that Qi Gong is enormously healing for the body, yet I am always amazed that it is so powerful. And if I had not seen it with my own eyes, I would have a hard time believing it. It is about ALS, a disease in which the muscles slowly deteriorate because the nerves harden and the stimuli do not come through anymore. The patients slowly lose their motoric skills in their hands and feet, end up in a wheelchair and die because of suffocation when the respiratory muscles stop working. With our patient you clearly see the deterioration of the muscles in his hands between thumb and forefinger. Instead of the usual flesh, his was only skin. On top of that the motoric skills of his other fingers were affected and his hands were always freezing cold. By doing a week of Qi

Gong exercises adapted to his situation and getting acupuncture several times, I saw his hands change. They got warmer, there was more movement in the fingers and the most magical thing of all was that the wells between thumb and index finger filled up. He himself is also impressed because he did not really believe that this practice could help him. I am really curious how his situation is going to evolve.

Unfortunately, I have no news. The person has returned to his homeland and his normal activities. He no longer could muster the courage to continue practicing Qi Gong. Especially in a degenerative disease you can not expect miracles to happen without changing your ways. Besides that, it's not easy for Westerners to go against regular medicine, to throw it overboard and to learn to rely on your own healing mechanisms. However painful, for yourself and your loved ones, death is inevitable. One with life. A life that, in the form of a Tibetan doctor, surprisingly revealed and solved my own subtle doubts

One of my Yoga Tree students asked me if I wanted to come to an introduction to Tibetan medicine given by his godson. To please him I went. I must admit that I was intrigued by what the doctor was telling. He could diagnose you by putting his fingertips on your wrist. I was curious what he could read in my pulse so I made an appointment with him. What did he see? There was so much wrong with me: I had a lot of mucus in my body, my stomach and uterus were cold (= not working optimally), my liver was fatty and my lungs contained too much phlegm. I had wind in my intestines and therefore suffer from indigestion. Tsjakka! Only my heart was perfectly healthy. Thank God for that one! Oh yes and Qi Gong had done a lot of good for my body. Can you guess what it would have been without? Death? My thoughts: About my womb, he was right, my periods come every month but last only two days and are rather stringy, lumpy and black instead of liquid and red. Making babies would be difficult. Really huh?! Luckily I don't want babies and got myself sterilized four years ago. I suppose he is right about my stomach because even with all the movement I have, I didn't lose weight (but didn't gain either). He advised me to drink a large glass of hot water first thing in the morning. That would help to make the stomach more warm and would also help with indigestion. Which I do not have by the way. Oops mistake! Now that glass of water doesn't seem to hurt me so I'll do that (test, test). Concerning my liver I can't think of anything but he could have had a point about the lungs. I have(?)/had exercise-induced asthma and yes sometimes I cough up mucus but I think that's more a consequence of the air pollution in Chiang Mai. Since I do Qi Gong, my way of breathing has changed so much that I no longer suffer from exercise-induced asthma. In the past I already started to wheeze when I had to cycle at a fast pace. Now no more, not even with the air pollution. So there I think he was wrong again. He also told me that a warm climate suited me better than a cold climate. I cannot agree more with that one.

Of course I talked about this experience with Ajahn. I wanted his opinion because I was a little startled. As I expected, he did not give me a straightforward answer. Instead he asked me how much value I attach to a pulse reading by someone who has seen me once. How much I dare to rely on my Qi Gong practice and my ever growing experience with what my body tells me. He also pointed out a contradiction in the diagnosis. According to the theory of the 5 elements, the liver has an effect on the heart, so an unhealthy liver and a healthy heart can't go together. Like in the case of too much cholesterol, which comes from the liver and affects the heart. Conclusion: it was intriguing to get to hear the doctor deducting all this from his three fingers on my wrists but due to my Qi Gong practice

I am much more in tune with my body. As a result, I know that he was mistaken on some points. He did not, in my opinion, give me a reason to worry. I think I'm doing a good job. That is what my body tells me and what I can rely on.

Qi Massage also strengthened that trust. Ajahn always insists on repetition, repetition and repetition. Flying time in his words. Participating in the same course a second time made me experience for myself what a progress I had made and how my body had become so much more sensitive. Or was the body always sensitive and was I not aware of it?

Qi Massage level 1. Although I followed that course last year, I got more out of it now. I more accurately sense the location of the points both within myself and within others. Which also means that I feel much better when they are not on it or when pressure is exerted by muscle strength (very painful). As a result, it was probably also much more tiring. We started every day at 9 am and did not finish before 6 pm. Long but interesting days!

Certainly interesting, also because I had many massages during my yoga training. Almost every week I went to a massage place. I needed these massages to relax my muscles because even yoga with all its stretching couldn't do that. And the stronger the massage the better. If it didn't hurt, it wasn't a good massage. I had to revise that opinion. A good massage doesn't have to hurt at all. A good massage helps your body to find its balance. Just like in Qi Gong practice. Qi Massage is an extra tool for this. Because of my own experience with yoga and Qi Gong I was very direct and judgemental when people asked me for my opinion about both. It came down to yoga is bad and Qi Gong is the best. Stop destroying your body with yoga, start practicing Qi Gong and everything will be fine. These days I'm more diplomatic in my answer. I believe that any movement system has its value. At a certain moment in a certain person's life. If only, as in my own case, to notice that it's not that. Although my wording has somewhat softened, I am still convinced that this form of Medical Qi Gong is something special. It can be practiced by everyone, whatever your state of health, whatever your age, whatever your prior knowledge may be. All that is needed is an open mind to not immediately refer to the trash concepts that are completely the opposite of what you have ever learned. And time. Time to transform the habits of a lifetime into new patterns. These new patterns in body and mind, unlike other methods, really help and heal you. I have seen that with my own eyes and experienced it within my own body.

L et me first tell you something about an insight that I got during the Yoga Tree class. All sorts of people come to that class, people who are on vacation and want to do some physical activity, people who are curious about Qi Gong, people who have physical problems and the last two or three weeks also people who have been doing yoga for several years or practice other styles of Qi Gong. At first sight they seem to be in perfect health until you to ask a bit further. They all have something. But mainly back and shoulder pains. In fact, I don't even have to ask anymore. When I see their posture, chest forward, shoulders backward, leaning slightly on the heels, I know enough. And it's confirmed time and again. I realize more and more what a jewel I found in this form of Medical Qi Gong. One that really does what it promises. Bringing back balance in the body. Someone with neck pain who has done a different style of Qi Gong for 5 years saying that after one hour of doing our exercises, something released in her neck is proof enough for me.

However things are not always that easy. Sometimes there is struggle, sometimes you need perseverance because all the injuries you have ever had come to say hello and go. Or stay a bit longer before they go. That's what is going on with my left knee this week. I really wondered where it came from and I had to go back a long way in my memory to a gymnastics gala more than 25 years ago. For reasons which I don't remember that knee was taped. A bit too firm so I fell off the beam a few times and felt really embarrassed. That injury came to say hello this week. To indicate that now is the time to finally treat it in the right way. To stimulate that weak spot, by finding the right way to move and stand. For sure, it's much easier to take a pill against the pain, but that is only a temporary solution. In the long run it only makes things worse. I am more for understanding my body (yes, I still have that scientific mind) and preferably without chemical junk. Isn't that why we are all here? To better understand ourselves? Both physically and mentally? Because just look at what goes on in your head when you are in pain! How strongly you resist the pain. And the more you want it to go away the worse it gets. The more you are in your head, the less you really feel what's going on in your body. If I am focussed on "Ugh, this hurts, I don't want this, why am I doing this again?" I can't sense that by adjusting my knee a little bit outward the pain eases. Head versus body! Your body doesn't lie, your head does! And we are so stuck in our heads that we don't even know that we lean too much backwards, that the knees fall in, the feet turn outwards, the shoulders are raised, the chest is tense, ... Resulting in all sorts of physical problems. Happy with this Qi Gong jewel that allows me to notice and change it!

Not only in The Yoga Tree I noticed what a jewel this Qi Gong method is, also at other times it dawned on me. Otherwise, 'my' students made me remember it.

A jahn has been in Jakarta for another five days and then it's my task to teach. Not always easy. Different levels, different characters, you can not do well for everyone. Maybe after 30+ years of experience like Ajahn but I don't even pretend to be at his level. Which doesn't mean that I don't learn a lot from it! Because of those experiences I grow both in my teaching and in my own practice. If I then get a work of art from one of my students with a very symbolic value, I can only be grateful for all that I witness and go through here.

Days became weeks and weeks became months. The April retreat in Bali and a subsequent holiday in Cambodia were a welcome change in the routine of every day. Slowly, almost unnoticeable a kind of resignation crept into my actions. Where at the beginning of the year I could be super excited about small things, I wondered more and more about what I was doing in the middle of the year. Qi Gong had become "work", no longer something that I enjoyed doing. I had the self-imposed idea that I should always show up, that I would miss something by being absent, that I would disappoint Ajahn by saying no. The straw that broke the camel's back was the realization that I tried to do good for everyone except for myself. I always encouraged students to listen carefully to their body and take rest when it asks rest. Sadly I forgot to listen to my own advice. It was time to change that. In the beginning I had a lot of trouble to say no. Today they have a four letter word for it: FOMO: fear of missing out. However, I stood my ground and it was the best gift I could have given myself.

What has become more important in the last month is more time for myself. I was fully committed to Qi Gong for the last two years, which meant that I was in the clinic every day, 7 days a week. It has brought me to where I am. I have grown enormously in my practice, in my teaching, in how I live. I can not be but grateful. Recently, however, it felt like I was out of balance (and Qi Gong is precisely about that), as if I had neglected a part of myself. The part that greatly enjoys a good book, the part that is creative, the part that likes to exchange ideas about all kinds of subjects, the part that likes to dance and go crazy. All those parts screamed for some attention but I ignored them. My body reacted. It indicated to have enough, it was exhausted, tired, listless. The moment I responded and decided to take Sunday off, everything got color again. Qi Gong became something to look forward to again, books were read instead of falling asleep over them, little creative projects that had been playing in my head for a while were finally undertaken, I went dancing. I feel that the different parts are slowly coming back into balance. Sometimes you have to experience some imbalance to reach balance. Sometimes you have to go through a period of "blah" to appreciate what "yeah" is. One can not do without the other. Isn't Life beautiful?

Life is indeed beautiful. By choosing myself I could be there again for others. I could again enjoy teaching and following classes. And I loved the fourth retreat in Bali.

Another retreat in Bali. The fourth. And if you ask me, the best so far. Little talking, a lot of practice. Don't question, don't think, just do it, again and again until it is right. Until your body got it. I thought it was wonderful.

What was also wonderful was that after more than 2 years I could finally take my parents to the clinic. To show them where and with what I filled my days. In addition to a few days practice there, we did all the touristy stuff. Not only in and around Chiang Mai but also in neighboring Cambodia. They came all the way to Thailand, I reckoned they should not miss Angkor Wat since it is so close. It was perhaps their only chance to visit this world heritage site. Time passed so quickly, before I realized it, 2016 was over and a new year had arrived.

9. IN SEARCH FOR A NEW BALANCE

After the visit of my parents, high season in the clinic started again. Students and instructors were returning, annual courses had to be given and new people were joining. I myself taught less and adopted again the role of student which gave me the opportunity to focus on my own practice. It also gave other instructor trainees the opportunity to start teaching and taught me to take a closer look at my own teaching. And then there was that one new patient I had a hard time with.

One of the new people is an ALS patient. He is at an advanced stage of the disease, which means he spends most of his day on a respirator. And the 'co-incidence' is that Ajahn has him assigned to me. That means that the patient and I are banned to the kitchen where we practice together. A very simplified version of the exercises because his condition doesn't allow him to do it in the normal way. Not easy at all and it really tires me out. First and foremost because he has a degenerative disease which causes his health to decline more every day, but also because of certain actions and believes, he doesn't make it any easier on himself. He comes to us to be helped but ignores the advice we give him. And then he's angry that things don't work. I understand that habits that have been around all your life are difficult to change, but in this kind of condition you would think it is easier. That you follow the advice of people who want you to function independently as long as possible. Yet I see a difference with the first time he came. He can do without his respirator for the time he's with us, which varies from 2 to 3 hours and his posture is less bent over, which only benefits his breathing. But I also see that his strength in his legs varies greatly from day to day, which means he sometimes can't stand up of his own accord and needs to be helped. It is an interesting case study, one that teaches me a lot but also one that exhausts me because I'm battling not only with his body but also with his mind. Nine out of ten, I'm in bed by nine on the days he's at the clinic. Yet I am grateful for the learning, because how often do you have the chance to see how someone deals with death approaching? Everyone is dying, that is a fact. We just don't want to see it, we don't believe it can be any moment. I see it as an invaluable life lesson to come into contact with someone who cannot but face it. But honestly, should I ever be confronted with similar circumstances, I hope that I can do it differently.

Was it due to the inevitability of his illness, or did the hustle and the bustle in the clinic have anything to do with it? The long days, the self-imposed idea that there was nothing more than Qi Gong? I started to question myself. And for the first time it really sunk in that any moment can be your last. Can I be really sure that I'll live tomorrow? If not, did I do everything I wanted to do? Did I see everything I wanted to see? All these musings made me want to sneak out. When Kathy asked me to go to Japan with her, I didn't hesitate for long. To leave everything behind for a while, no Qi Gong, no ALS patient, just go around and have fun. And that was what I needed to realize that I really put my heart and soul into Qi Gong. That realization came during an informal teaching moment with a friend of Kathy. I had come along to support her, not to teach myself. But as it goes, things ran differently than planned and I ended up teaching half of the class. At that moment it dawned on me: "Actually, I like to do this. In fact, it is great to be able to help people this way." At that moment I also decided last minute to participate in the 5th retreat in Bali. Admittedly only the second week because the first week I was invited to a wedding in Cambodia. While in Cambodia, there were a number of teaching moments seemingly coming out of nowhere, strengthening my belief that I could not throw Qi Gong overboard. That it was far too valuable. I just had to find a different rhythm. One that allowed me to do other fun things besides Qi Gong. Or just do nothing. While after the retreat in the clinic the normal rhythm was resumed, I left the teaching more and more to the other instructors. I felt that their time had come and that my time to explore other places had arrived. That feeling was magnified when halfway through 2017 I got rid of all my diaries. Sixteen notebooks which harboured all my impressions, emotions and adventures of the past three years and half. It was like a weight lifted off my shoulders. I felt so light. The past was where it belonged, in the garbage bin. I was finished with it. And ready and open for something different. When out of the blue there was a possibility to go teaching in Cambodia, I did not hesitate. It was the right time to share all the knowledge and experience I gained during my time at the clinic and to share with others the power of this system. 3 years, 3 months and 13 days of heights and lows, of wonder and overwhelm, of love and suffering, but especially of infinite gratitude. Gratitude for the knowledge and the patience that Ajahn brings up for me and his other students, every day again. Gratitude for the lessons of life gained, for the wisdom that has nested in my heart. Gratitude for the chances and opportunities that I've received, for the people who believed in me and are still doing so. Gratitude for the support, friendship and openness of students. I may have left Chiang Mai, the ties with Ajahn and the TQH community remain strong. Qi Gong is in my blood now.

MORE WANDER AND WONDER

My wanderings are continuing. After an intermezzo in Cambodia I have now landed in Sitia, Crete where I am available to introduce you to the secrets of Medical Qi Gong. Do you dare to start your own wander to wonder? My miracle path can only stay a miracle if there are people who, together with me, dare to take the road to a new way of moving. The first step, one email, one phone call or one message you have to take yourself. We will finish the rest of the road together. Looking forward to it!

Ils

qiflowqigong@gmail.com
www.qiflowqigong.com/contact
www.facebook.com/qigonginsitia
via whatsapp: +30 6948 69 22 67

ACKOWNLEDGEMENTS

To Life that has been given to me by my parents.
To those same parents who always let me go my own way.
To my brother and his family
To my friends
To Ajahn and the TQH community
To my students
To all other amazing living beings that are part of my world.

Thousand times thanks

ABOUT THE AUTHOR

As a child, born and raised in a small village in Belgium, Ils wanted to become a researcher. She studied Pharmacy at the University of Ghent, where she also obtained her PhD in Microbiology after an extra master's year in Biotechnology at KU Leuven. After various jobs that were not fulfilling, she decided to take a sabbatical year. She went to Asia where she discovered Medical Qi Gong. Ils gave her life a new direction and went deep into the age-old wisdom of this system. During that process she also began teaching. First in the clinic under the supervision of her teacher, later, after 9 months also in The Yoga Tree, a dance and yoga center in the heart of Chiang Mai. She stayed with her teacher for more than 3 years where she practiced, taught and worked with patients with all kinds of disorders. She also assisted her teacher with acupuncture and she herself gave Qi Massages. After about 5000 hours of Medical Qi Gong practice and teaching, she felt it was time to share the Qi Gong way with everyone who wants to take their health and their lives into their own hands. To learn more about the in and outs please visit www.qiflowqigong.com.

Ils Cools